Conquer Chronic Pain

Conquer Chronic Pain

An Innovative Mind-Body Approach

PETER PRZEKOP, DO, PHD

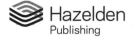

Hazelden
Publishing

Hazelden Publishing
Center City, Minnesota 55012
hazelden.org/bookstore

Library of Congress Cataloging-in-Publication Data

Przekop, Peter, 1954-
    Conquer chronic pain : an innovative mind-body approach / Peter Przekop.
      pages cm
    ISBN 978-1-61649-789-7 (paperback)
1. Chronic pain—Alternative treatment. 2. Mind and body therapies.
3. Medicine, Psychosomatic. I. Title.
    RB127.P79 2015
    616'.0472—dc23

                              2015023099

Editor's note
The names, details, and circumstances may have been changed to protect the
privacy of those mentioned in this publication.
    This publication is not intended as a substitute for the advice of health
care professionals.

19 18 17 16 15   1 2 3 4 5 6

Cover design: Theresa Jaeger Gedig
Interior design and typesetting: Terri Kinne, Trina Christensen
Interior illustrations: John P. Hearst
Developmental editor: Sid Farrar
Production editor: Heather Silsbee

*To Allison, who is beautiful and remains
one of a kind, and to our son, Kojo.*

Contents

Acknowledgments

There are many people I would like to thank who have contributed to the ideas that went into this book. First and foremost, all of the patients with whom I have interacted who have endured and contributed to my development. To my parents and family—Marylou, Bun, Jayne, Kal, and Trixie. To Chet, Oscar, Tom, Otis, Phoebe, Sasha, Ted, Trina, Ziggy, and Joe. Also Jay, Doug, Tom, Jim, Joe, Anis, Said, Billy, Mark, Gisela, Bill, Jim, John, and Bob. And to all of those people I have not mentioned who have been instrumental in my development or lack of it.

Many thanks also to Vince Hyman, Sid Farrar, and Heather Silsbee for editing and support throughout the process. And to J. P. Hearst for his artwork and Liz Kipp and Allison for editorial support.

Introduction

I believe that no one is born to suffer. I also believe that your brain, mind (which I define as our ability to represent what is directly before us, recall what we have experienced, and imagine what may occur in the future), and body all have the ability to heal. If you are suffering from chronic pain, this book is my best attempt to help you do this because you—and everyone else—deserve it. I want to do my part to end that suffering.

Many of the ideas in this book will at first seem counterintuitive. We learn about pain early in life. Touch a hot stove—pain. Bump yourself—pain. So we are accustomed to the idea that pain is associated with a specific injury.

This is true for short-term (acute) pain. But when pain persists for months, something different is going on. That is where the counterintuitive aspect occurs.

I have devoted my career as a physician to treating chronic pain. The patients with whom I work have grown used to the daily experience of pain. Yet the source of their pain remains a mystery. Unlike the child who bumps her head, my patients (and often other people who have treated them) truly do not understand why they continue to have pain despite receiving treatment. They usually have been told that it has to do with an injury in some part of their body—some damage, some inflammation, some wound—that is as yet unresolved.

But there is a curious thing about chronic pain. Many doctors, myself included, have observed that some people with a similar pathology (the same condition) do not continue to have physical pain after receiving the appropriate treatment for that condition. For example, one person may experience chronic pain as a result of a neck injury, while the pain subsides after a reasonable amount of time for another person with the same injury. Why would these two people have such different experiences? Why does one feel miserable, while the other feels great?

The full answer to this question is still being explored by chronic pain clinicians and researchers, but I, along with many other medical professionals, have come to believe that part of the answer is that the pain is, in a very real sense, "in your brain." There is strong evidence that the experience of chronic pain happens in your brain, and the way you interpret signals from your body to your brain is shaped by your very unique *mind*. This makes the experience of pain different for every person.

That is what I mean when I say that the ideas in this book may seem counterintuitive. This book is not about helping you "fix" the place you think your pain originates from—your neck or your back or your joints or your hip. This book is about *you*, the whole "brain-mind-body" you. That is why my goal in writing this book is to help you understand the vicious cycle of chronic pain so you can retrain your brain, mind, *and* body to break that cycle.

I have included exercises that will help you develop your own insight into how and why your brain-mind-body feels chronic pain. I will start

PLEASE TAKE NOTE

If you are suffering from chronic pain and what you have been doing to treat it has not been working, this book offers you an approach that has produced positive results for hundreds of people. The ideas and exercises in this book are not meant to replace your doctor's treatment plan if that has been helpful. Rather, this book is designed to give you additional tools to supplement what you are already doing, assuming the two approaches are compatible, or to offer an alternative approach to explore if what you have been doing has not provided relief over time.

However, this, or any other approach, will not be effective if you do not follow the recommended procedures consistently and thoroughly, as long as you are not experiencing any negative reactions. You should discontinue any treatment approach, including practicing the exercises in this book, if you find that your condition is worsening. In that case, you should stop what you are doing and seek professional help.

in the first chapter with my own journey, from a student curious about the mind to my work as a physician helping people in chronic pain. My journey has been about being inquisitive, listening to and learning from people like you, doing research, and trying new things with my patients based on what I have found to help them heal.

In this book, you will learn what I and other researchers have been discovering over the last ten years: that the conditions that prepare us to experience chronic physical pain may begin long before we actually feel physical pain and may involve emotional or social pain. As you read on, you will understand what I mean by this and why this is the case.

> Take "S.," for example. When I met S. she had debilitating pain that restricted her to a wheelchair. For the first two weeks I worked with her, she did not understand that the pain she was experiencing in her body actually began many years before, probably when she was a child, as an entirely different, non-physical type of pain. Her pain occurred because she had been the victim of severe adversity, having been both emotionally and sexually abused. She had no idea that these adverse events had set the tone for a future life of debilitating pain. Once she uncovered the links between her past, how she truly felt, and how she held those feelings and memories inside of her body, brain, and mind, she was able to practice some activities that helped her change her life, step out of her wheelchair, and free herself from pain physically, mentally, and spiritually. Until she experienced it, she thought life without pain was impossible.

Through activities such as the ones you will learn in this book, S. learned to venture inside of her brain-mind-body and feel things that she had never felt before, process them, and free herself from their burden. I know that S.'s story may sound implausible, perhaps a bit like the old miracle-healing gimmicks you once found in the back of cheap magazines or on late-night television. But in the past two years, I have observed sixty-one other wheelchair-bound patients reduce their pain and leave their wheels behind. I have seen over five hundred other people dramatically reduce their pain by using the same type of exercises that appear in this book.

The foundation of my work and this book is the belief, based on my clinical work and research, that much of what leads people to chronic pain is a combination of the following:

- their past experience
- how they dealt with that experience
- their present stressors
- their *cognitive style,* or the way they think and process information

As you read through this book, you will learn more about these key ideas and what they have to do with freeing yourself from chronic pain.

My Goals for Your Journey

There are two parts to this book. Part 1 is informational. You will learn about the nature of chronic pain, the structure of the brain, how the mind is different from the brain and how the mind works, and how the functions of brain and mind are changed by the experience of chronic pain. You will consider a question that might seem provocative at first: *How is chronic pain like addiction?* You will also learn, on an intellectual level, how releasing past adversity and negative experiences can help your brain, mind, and body return to a positive state. Learning this information is vital to your recovery, but the way to overcome chronic pain is not through the intellect alone. Much of recovery occurs through adopting practices that activate your body's natural healing abilities. Part 2 consists of eighteen exercises that help you accomplish this. A few of the exercises involve movement, but most of them are designed to help you venture inward, where real healing begins.

After reading this book, you will clearly understand how I think chronic pain should be defined and you will have a new perspective of the current state of treatment for chronic pain in the United States, the level of widespread suffering, and the problems caused by many of the current treatment methods. As you read through the chapters, you will also gain a basic understanding of how the brain works. You will see that, contrary to what you may have assumed or heard in the past, your brain has the ability to constantly change. You will learn about this thing we call *mind* and its ability to somehow represent reality as almost a movie being played out in our heads. Further, you will see how this capacity to represent the world can be an amazingly helpful thing, or a very harmful experience when the "movie" becomes negative and the negativity repeats itself.

If you are currently experiencing chronic pain, you will gain insight into beliefs that may be keeping you in a state of suffering. You will understand how chronic stress and other factors—such as the inability to feel, difficulty processing emotions, and ineffective coping skills—contribute to the experience of chronic pain. You will see how your *autobiographical narrative,* the story you tell yourself about your own life, affects the way you experience things every day. You will understand that your narrative interacts with your moment-to-moment memory (the *working memory* that helps you understand your life) to influence your experience of pain. Finally, you will learn that without mind and perception, there is no pain, and that without the judgment of pain as more than a sensation or energy, there would be no suffering.

I realize these ideas may sound radical and they may not make sense to you at this point. However, as you read on you will see that there is a logic to these ideas that can lead you to better understand and completely change how you experience your chronic pain. The exercises and background in the book hold the potential to change your life. My goal for you from reading this book is the same as it is with my patients: that you dramatically reduce your relationship with pain.

• • •

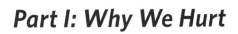

Part I: Why We Hurt

1

Learning from My Patients

Not everyone who has a particular injury goes on to have chronic pain. Only a small subset does. That is one of many fascinating mysteries about chronic pain, and it is why I became so intrigued with chronic pain as the focus of my work. I wanted to know what it was about that subset of individuals that led them to have persistent pain. More important, I wanted to know how I could reverse it.

About ten years ago I began seeing patients with chronic pain in an outpatient clinic. They were but a few of the some 100 million people who suffer from chronic pain in the United States. (Worldwide there are 1.5 billion people with chronic pain.) Their cases were quite a challenge—and I seldom back away from a challenge!

I decided to collect more information. I gathered as many patients with severe chronic pain as I could find, all of whom had failed traditional therapy and all of whom were at the point where they felt they had no alternatives. Some wanted to die. They were absolutely helpless and hopeless. To learn more, on Monday nights I assembled them in the waiting room of a private practice traditional pain clinic and invited my wife, a pediatric neurologist, to attend the meeting. I began the first meeting by encouraging the patients to speak. I simply allowed them to tell each other the story of their journey and of their present misery.

These patients' stories showed how difficult their problems had been. Hearing their experiences was very informative. As I listened to them, I began to realize that all of these people had been in pain long before the onset of the physical pain. Yet each one honestly thought that no one else could understand them, that their journey was unique, and that somehow they had been left behind to suffer alone.

Prior to this meeting, they apparently had been asked only about their symptoms and levels of pain. This meeting seemed to be the first time they were given the opportunity to tell their whole stories to other people who would listen to what the pain meant to them, not just what their symptoms were and what level of pain they felt on a scale of 1 to 10—a common question health care professionals use to gauge the severity of pain. Slowly, just by the process of telling their stories, they began the healing process. Here are a few examples of what they shared.

> There was "M.," who had been in pain for more than two decades. The chronic, widespread pain she felt all over her body had decimated her social life. She had not felt close to anyone in years and had come to the point of thinking about suicide on many occasions. She had seen more doctors and tried more pills than she could count. M. believed that no one understood her pain, that no one understood the depths of her despair. When she began to disclose it, she saw that others in the room were able to easily relate. This opened the door to her healing.
>
> ———
>
> There was "V.," a busy woman with three children, a career, aging parents who seemed to need her help, and a brother with special needs whom she visited several times a week. V. had been feeling deep and ever-increasing pain across her hips and lower back for two years. Yet she stoically persisted. She did not want her family to know how much her pain was affecting her because she was afraid she would let them down. She was afraid they would see her as a bad wife, a negligent mother, a disloyal sister, and an insensitive daughter.
>
> ———
>
> There was "D.," a veteran of the Vietnam War who never told anyone about his combat experience. D. had pain in every joint of his body. He had no idea that his fears, the things he witnessed, and the combat memories he had hidden inside were dramatically contributing to his pain until he began to disclose the emotions that he held for decades.

I was amazed at what could be done simply by giving chronic pain patients an open forum to discuss their stories. More people began to come to the group. I became convinced that beyond any specific diagnosis these patients were given, they had a distinct disease called *chronic pain*.

I was not always nice to them. I pushed them to explore more of what they held inside, what emotions they were experiencing, and what feelings they were trying to avoid or repress. I realized that they had been told they were ill for so long that they had, in a sense, *become the disease*.

"T." is an excellent example. He had chronic daily headaches. He would come into the meeting room, sit in a chair, hold his head, and lean forward with his eyes closed. He was certain that he was always going to have headaches and that there was no hope. I realized that his case fit the typical profile of chronic daily headaches that can become extraordinarily debilitating. They often begin as either tension-type headaches or migraine headaches, and they can actually be made worse through the use of certain medications such as opioids, triptans, or non-steroidal anti-inflammatory medications that are prescribed to treat them. He had seen multiple providers for help, and it occurred to me that he had somehow lost himself in the description of the disease process—that the chronic headaches had become a pivotal part of T.'s identity and that he had lost touch with who he really was beyond the pain.

I began to wonder whether the perception of the pain and how it almost merged with one's personal identity was actually part of the disease process of chronic pain. I even started calling members of the group by their individual diseases instead of their names. Over time some of them began to understand that I was doing this to show that they were contributing to their chronic pain state by over-identifying with it.

Most of these patients had previously been prescribed opioids to deal with their pain. Opioids are synthetic or semisynthetic narcotic drugs similar to opiates, such as morphine, which are derived from the poppy seed. Well-known opioids include oxycodone, hydrocodone, and heroin. They are beneficial drugs when used to quell short-term pain and for some other purposes. But with long-term use, the brain changes in response to these drugs, becoming more tolerant of the effects and requiring larger doses to achieve the same results. They also have undesirable side effects and, when misused, can lead to addiction. (In chapter 3, you will learn about the current epidemic of painkiller abuse and overdose, and how this relates to the way we have been medicating chronic pain.)

I was able to get most of these patients to detoxify from their prescribed opioids and other addictive medications. They were absolutely terrified at first, and they were reluctant to give up their drugs. But I had become convinced that there was no healing to be done while their brains were being altered by an addictive substance.

After working with this group, I wanted to gather more information. I have been trained to do research in the basic sciences, but I had never done research with human clinical populations, so at first I stumbled. Research on humans is very different from research that is done in the basic sciences, so I had to learn quickly. But eventually I was able to gather meaningful information. I began by giving a survey to over 560 people who were presenting for their initial evaluation at a chronic pain clinic. One of the questions I asked was, "If you had to go on as you are now with this pain or had the choice of death, which one would you choose?" Over 54 percent of the people who responded said they would choose death. After the survey, this same group was placed on opioid pain medications for over six months. After that time I surveyed them again. If the pain treatment was making their lives better, you would expect the percentage choosing death would decrease dramatically. Quite the opposite happened: six months later the percentage of people who would choose death had risen to 68 percent.

Something was wrong with our approach to treating chronic pain!

This information only strengthened my growing opinion that current treatments for pain that seek to numb symptoms or stop pain were inadequate. I went on to read much of the research on chronic pain. I found confirmation for my belief that chronic pain is a disease in and of itself— a disease of the brain. At first that seems counterintuitive because, on examination and by report of patients with chronic pain, it is certain areas of the body that hurt. Those areas were associated with a diagnosable disease, and those areas were where the patient perceived the pain. However, after going on to read many more articles and having seen many more patients, I clearly saw that there was a complex relationship among where it hurts, what the pathology in that area may or may not be, the level of pain, and the amount of disability caused by that pain.

The most dramatic example I have seen of this occurred when I was a neurology resident in the emergency room. There I saw a patient whose spine had degenerated so much that he could not move from midchest down because his spine had essentially collapsed onto his spinal cord. I asked this gentleman if he had ever experienced pain. He said no. Yet I had seen many examples of people with minimal or no abnormalities in their spine who felt dramatic pain. I had also read a case report of a person who, from birth, was unable to experience pain—because of a condition that altered a sodium channel in the nervous system that is responsible for the perception of pain—and yet during the extreme stress of the loss of a loved one, this person developed a headache. This meant that extreme emotional stress was able to cause pain *even though the person did not have the physiological capability to experience pain.* This example indicated to me that clearly something else must be going on. I saw that many physicians had taken the common treatment for acute pain—for example, opioid medications—and applied it to chronic pain. While this approach was fine for acute pain, the evidence was growing that it did not necessarily work for chronic pain.

The question then became, If chronic pain is in fact a brain disease, how do you treat the *brain* of someone with this disease? This raised several additional questions:

- When meeting new patients, how do you convince them that what they have is a disease of the brain?
- How do you explain that chronic pain *is a disease in itself* that must be treated?
- Further, how do you help patients see that this disease of chronic pain may have little or nothing to do with the pathology that they

have been told they have or that has shown up on blood tests, imaging studies, or physical exams?

The Roots of My Journey

The roots of my journey toward trying to understand chronic pain probably began as an undergraduate college student. I was not a particularly good student—I was more interested in sports than academics. But somewhere along the line, I developed an intense curiosity about the relationships between brain, mind, and body. At first it seemed intuitively obvious that there was a relationship between brain, mind, and body and that somehow all of consciousness was the result of the actions of the brain. (I will explain shortly my definition of the difference between the mind and the brain.) The more I learned, the more gaps in knowledge were created, and the relationship that I thought was obvious became less clear. The philosopher David Hume wrote about the phenomenon that as knowledge increases, it often creates more gaps in what we know. Hume's was probably one of the best lessons I learned, in that it made me even more inquisitive and motivated to add to my knowledge.

I also had become fascinated by the relationship between consciousness and spirituality. From a young age, I had always wondered if there was something unique about humans that would allow us to realize our potential for well-being—some sort of an inner energy or power that would bring about healing if we could only tap into it. I knew on some level that any manifestation of this healing process would have to come from within and that tapping into it was going to require a search inward instead of outward. This belief is one of the foundations of what is ahead in this book: if we learn to balance the amount of stress that we hold, our chances of healing will dramatically improve. At first this statement sounds very unscientific. However, as you read on, you will learn that this idea is indeed supported by evidence.

I realized that determining how to go about this inward search would require that I understand more about the nature of consciousness. We have within us the ability to represent what is directly before us, recall what we have experienced, and imagine what may occur in the future.

All of this occurs in a place we call *mind.* Somehow mind is related to the structure and function of our brain. Understanding this relationship was key to figuring out why some individuals are able to heal after an injury yet others go on to develop chronic pain. I began to ask, "Is chronic pain something that has occurred in the brain, the mind, the body, or all three?" The research I studied told me that indeed it may be in our brain and mind, and it may be heavily impacted by past experience. I became increasingly interested in the brain and the mind, and how they function normally and in the face of disease.

After some postgraduate studies at McGill University, I decided to pursue a master's degree in clinical psychology. As part of my master's degree program in the mid-1980s, I conducted a research experiment that showed that the outer layer of the brain, which is called the cortex, was able to serve multiple functions. For example, the area of the brain that helps produce language also plays a role in the movement of one's right finger. So, if you speak and move your finger at the same time, there is a decrease in performance of both hand movement and speech. This finding taught me that the brain has the ability to take on many tasks at once but that if overlapping areas are active at the same time, there is a decrease in overall performance. We all can observe this phenomenon whenever we see a person trying to talk on a cell phone and drive a car at the same time!

I then became interested in neurobiology and was able to pursue a PhD in that discipline. My major interest was in how alterations in the environment could change the normal development of the brain. I learned that normal brain development could be altered—that is, the structure and function could change—as early as in utero by changes in the environment. The brain, however, retained the ability to normalize its structure and function when normal conditions were restored. This capacity of the brain to change is called *neuroplasticity.* The basis of the treatments that will be explained later in this book is the direct result of these experiments and those of many other researchers, which have shown that when the brain is given optimal environmental stimulation, it can normalize—that is, return to its normal functioning—and this ability is retained throughout one's lifetime.

Before these experiments we did not think the brain's ability to change continued throughout a lifetime. In 1967, Eric Lenneberg, a pioneering researcher on the topics of language acquisition and cognitive psychology, demonstrated that at age twelve the brain was fixed and did not retain the ability to change. This was based on his experiments showing that children who had undergone brain surgery that removed the part of the cortex responsible for language production were not able to produce perfectly normal speech for the rest of their lives.

However, subsequent studies have shown that we retain the ability to change our brain long into our lives. This ability does decline with age, but it is always there. This research gave me hope, since it suggested that many diseases of the brain that formerly were thought to be permanent might actually be alterable. We now know that Lenneberg had demonstrated the concept of a *sensitive period* in brain development. In essence, during this sensitive period of development, the brain can be more influenced by environmental stimulation than at other times. Lenneberg's studies led people to believe that after the sensitive period was over, the brain was no longer able to change. In fact, it was assumed that it had lost all plasticity. This assumption has been proven to be not completely true.

Eventually I continued on to earn a PhD, but I realized I wanted to pursue further education and work directly with people. I chose osteopathic medicine, an alternative medical approach emphasizing the manipulation of the muscle tissue and bones, so I could do whole person care and use my hands with osteopathic manipulation to attempt to heal people. On the first day of school I was lucky enough to meet a student who is now my wife. This changed my life and my practice completely; it was she who helped me better understand the role of the mind in chronic pain and who gave me the skills I would need to develop alternative treatments for people with chronic pain. She showed me how to refine my ability to use my hands to gather information about patients and then use energy to help those patients heal.

As a third-year medical student, I began to work with patients. The first day of seeing patients I was nervous and did not know what to expect. I was not sure how to interview people to get needed facts, but soon realized all I had to do was be myself. It also became clear that I was the only student who wanted to see the patients with chronic pain—my colleagues and mentors were happy when they did not have to see these patients. As I got to know these patients, I learned that they had much more than just chronic physical pain and were among the most complex and miserable people I had ever been around. Moreover, their treatment plans were failing them, and they wanted to begin down a new road that would bring them toward healing.

I was determined to find a way to bring them hope and relief. I realized that we needed a novel approach to chronic pain—a way that would treat the whole person. I decided to take on that challenge.

A Vision of Healing from Chronic Pain

After graduating from medical school, I was uncertain what additional training would be best to enable me to begin a career treating people with chronic pain. I completed an internship in internal medicine and thereafter a short period of training in neurology, and then finished in internal medicine, reasoning that internal medicine training would give me a broad spectrum of knowledge from which to approach these very complex patients.

I ended up doing a fellowship in addiction medicine and soon after added a six-month extension in chronic pain. I had a vision of developing a way to treat patients who were experiencing chronic pain and comorbid diseases, such as substance use disorders, depression, and anxiety, using non-pharmacologic techniques. The first job I had involved making house calls to patients who were too ill to go to a doctor's office. In this position, I focused on improving my skills in interacting with patients and in trying to identify the underlying causes of their chronic diseases.

It was becoming apparent to me that many people become chronically ill because of their lifestyle, management of emotions, and coping strategies. I found that people who are unable to cope with chronic stress, people who internalize emotions, and those who avoided feeling anything that they held inside had an increased tendency to become chronically ill. Those people who had experienced some extraordinarily adverse event, such as abuse or a bad accident, and had not adequately coped with that experience also had more of a tendency to become chronically ill. I began to wonder whether certain people were more likely to develop chronic pain and whether the pain experienced by the people I worked with involved chronic stress or an experience of adversity. That was when I also began to wonder if there was a *disease* called chronic pain that was independent from all other diagnoses that involve pain. Were certain people predisposed to chronic pain because of the way their past experiences and the effects of these stressful experiences interacted with alterable genetic material?

I realized that chronic pain was often viewed as essentially untreatable, with only symptom relief possible at best. This model where only the symptoms were treated was causing many people with chronic pain to identify with the disease they had been diagnosed with and, to some extent, to describe and present themselves in terms of that disease. I became even more convinced that the proper treatment of pain, therefore, must involve helping the person remember any adverse event in his or her past, any inability to cope, and anything else that weakened their ability to properly process stress and emotions. If these underlying roots were not properly addressed and treated, I concluded, we would only be treating the symptoms instead of the possible causes of chronic pain. This is when I realized how complex the problem would be, but also that there may be a novel solution. What held people back from realizing their full potential could be negative events from their past, and these same negative events could be contributing to their development of chronic pain.

My next opportunity to develop my approach came when I was offered a job as the medical director of an addiction rehabilitation center. They had a pain program that was directed by someone who soon became a trusted friend and colleague, someone who had been in Twelve Step recovery for over thirty years.* The rehabilitation center was cautious about my approach, and I had to do much of my work on my own, but as the patients began to respond, I was on the road to formulating the unique

---

* The Twelve Steps were originally developed by Alcoholics Anonymous (AA) in their textbook of the same name to give alcoholics a structured program of practicing their recovery along with attending peer support meetings. This recovery model was eventually adopted by Al-Anon for family members of alcoholics and by groups recovering from other addictions, including Narcotics Anonymous (NA), Gamblers Anonymous (GA), and many others. Many addiction treatment programs also use the Twelve Steps as a part of their treatment protocols.

treatment method I had envisioned to deal with both substance use disorders and chronic pain.

After two years at that job I was asked to start a pediatric chronic pain and headache clinic at Loma Linda University Medical School. I am still at this job, and it has been a dramatic and rewarding learning experience. Soon after that, I was also invited to develop a chronic pain program at the Betty Ford Center. This was my first opportunity to fully develop a program based on my research and patient successes. I have been there for almost five years as of this writing, and we have helped over five hundred people with chronic pain and addiction to achieve successful recovery from both disorders. Ninety-six percent of people leave our chronic pain program pain free. The average amount of pain that people arrive with is 7.2 out of 10 (with 0 being pain free and 10 being excruciating pain). They leave the program with an average score of .06—close to no pain at all. After one year, three out of four (74 percent) report that they are still doing well. I am happy with these results but I believe we can continue to improve the program and achieve even better outcomes.

From My Journey to Yours

I have told you about my personal journey so that you can see how my observations, experiences, and most important, my patients have shaped a non-pharmacologic approach to treating chronic pain. Of course, the goal of this book is to help people with chronic pain follow these same methods. But it is important that you learn about the nature of chronic pain and the functions of the brain before you begin trying the exercises I use in my program. My patients have told me that they have benefited from learning about the following:

- how the brain works
- how chronic pain works in the brain
- how the opioid pain medications that are commonly prescribed for pain affect these brain processes
- how the mind works and how it is different from the brain
- how the brain, mind, and body work together to make us who we are and enable us to create our own unique experience of pain

In the next chapter, you will begin this journey by learning about the nature of chronic pain.

• • •

2

Understanding Chronic Pain

In this chapter, you will learn an alternative definition for chronic pain—one that differs from most clinical definitions. This definition helps you understand how any pain experienced throughout your lifetime, whether mental or physical, can affect your present physical pain. As you will see, past experiences and the impact they have on how you process current information (sensations, thoughts, and emotions) can pave the road to chronic pain. The process that leads to chronic pain often begins long before you experience any physical pain or have it diagnosed by a doctor.

You will also learn about the current treatments for chronic pain—some of which you may have experienced—and how these treatments tend to focus on symptoms rather than on the person and the underlying issues that may predispose a person to chronic physical pain. As briefly noted in the last chapter, medical treatments for chronic pain have been borrowed from approaches that have been successful in treating acute (short-term) pain. These strategies often fail when they are applied to chronic pain because chronic pain is a different disease and, therefore, must be treated differently than acute pain. As a result, some medical treatments for chronic pain do not bring long-term relief to the patient and can actually intensify the patient's level of pain.

How Many of Us Are Hurting?

Chronic pain affects as many as 30 percent of Americans. You do not have to like math to understand that 30 percent is a large portion of the population. In fact, it is *huge*. Think about it this way: every time you go out and are in a large enough group of people, it is likely that one out of every three have chronic pain. As you read this, there are about

320 million people living in the United States, which means that approximately 110 million of them are likely to have chronic pain. So you can see, we have a big problem in this country. But chronic pain is a worldwide problem. Estimates are that about 15 to 20 percent of people in the United States experience it as a serious and debilitating condition. That is a smaller number, but still huge. It means that in the United States, 50 to 65 million people may have serious, long-lasting pain that has a dramatic effect on their lives. This pain is often so severe that it changes their lives. It damages their ability to feel whole, to relate to partners, parents, or co-workers. It makes life's daily demands a tough struggle. And the economic costs are about $600 billion per year in the United States alone.

Tragically, our current medical treatments are, for the most part, inadequate and offer only partial relief. We spend a lot of money trying to help, but the true cost of chronic pain is seen in the effect it has on those who suffer from it and on their families, colleagues, and society as a whole. Unless you have experienced it, you may not be able to imagine the depths of hopelessness and despair some people with chronic pain experience.

The Meaning of Chronic Pain

The accepted definition of *chronic pain* among health care professionals and researchers who treat and study patients is "any pain that persists for three months or more." This definition is nonspecific and somewhat vague, since most people over the age of forty would seem to qualify. As will become clear when you read on, chronic pain is much more than just the sensation of pain. It is more about how one defines pain and how severe it is, as well as how long it persists. As chronic pain progresses, it can take on more and more meaning in one's life.

Two people can have knee pain. One is able to adequately deal with the pain and it has little effect on that person's life. Another person may be in constant agony with pain severe enough to dramatically affect this person's life. Yet, both people have chronic pain. The first person is on the low end of a pain continuum, the end that represents the least severity of chronic pain. This level of pain causes suffering, but it is manageable. The second person is on the opposite end of the pain continuum, where there is overwhelming suffering.

It is important to understand that once pain becomes chronic, the sensation of pain is not the most important aspect of pain. Rather, the person's *interpretation* of that pain is what has the most dramatic effect. It is also important to understand that people with any kind of chronic pain must take care of themselves. Without adequate treatment, such as the approach that will be described in this book, even pain that appears manageable can eventually take over one's life and have a dramatic negative effect.

These observations have led me to define chronic pain differently from the traditional definition. Please read the definition below and take a moment to really think it through:

> *Chronic pain* is any sensation with a negative context in the mind that is holding one from being able to heal.

I have chosen this definition based on the belief that any sensation within the body connected with a negative emotion can be interpreted as pain. Thus, whenever you feel emotional pain, it always has a physical component and, if unaddressed, it can stop you from being able to heal. I believe it can also have a dramatic effect on the future experience of chronic pain, in that the more emotional pain you feel in your body, the more susceptible you become to developing chronic pain.

This belief is based on studies that have shown that all bodily sensations perceived as negative (that is, as painful) are processed through the same neural pathways. It is only when this pain stops being simply a sensory event and, through a neural pathway in the brain, is *interpreted* as pain in the mind that we attach a story to it. As briefly described in the introduction, our mind has a constant, ongoing narrative—a kind of internal story or "movie"—that is much more than just a sensory event. It occurs in parallel to what the brain processes. The mind interprets the sensation of pain and gives it a social, emotional, or physical context, or story. In other words, as the brain processes information, it *does not care* what caused the pain or what type of pain it is. All painful sensations are processed through the same neural pathways in the brain. It is our *mind* that attaches past experience to the pain and interprets it.

The important thing to remember about the brain is that as certain pathways are used more and more, they strengthen and become easier to stimulate with weaker signals. It is like going to the gym to strengthen a muscle through repetitive exercise. In the same way, you strengthen pathways in the brain through repetitive use. This is why I say that the experience of pain throughout your lifetime may influence the development of chronic physical pain, as the pain pathways are strengthened through repetitive use. The neuroscientist Donald Hebb was the first to describe this phenomenon, which he called *cell assembly*. That is, as connected nerve cells in the brain are repeatedly stimulated, they assemble into pathways that gain strength with more stimulation. Chapter 6 on neuroplasticity explains this in more detail.

The good news is that you can change these pathways. When given enriched environmental stimulation, the body and brain can heal. You will be learning about this throughout this book and especially in the exercises in part 2, but the lesson begins with learning these facts about your brain.

You will note that my definition of chronic pain differs in some important ways from the more accepted version of "any pain that persists for three months or more." I believe that my definition is probably more meaningful. I have developed it for the purposes of the treatment methods contained in this book, so let us investigate it a bit more.

I say chronic pain is "any sensation with a negative context" because we have a tendency to think that chronic pain has to be physical; that is, it has to reside in some specific areas of our body and be associated with tissue damage. However, if you reflect on your past negative emotional experiences, you will likely remember that these emotions usually had a physical component as well. It is not without meaning that we say we have a "broken heart" when we lose a loved one, whether through death or betrayal. The experience is emotional, but we feel it physically, often in our chest. Or consider anyone who has had symptoms of depression or anxiety. These problems have a physical component that can be perceived as pain—feelings of deep heaviness, weakness, or being dragged down when depressed, or feelings of jittery vibration when experiencing anxiety, such as the sensation of "butterflies in my stomach."

The more of these experiences we have had at an earlier age, the better we have prepared the neural networks (or, as Hebb stated, the cell assembly) for future pain.

> Consider my patient "C." who developed interstitial cystitis (chronic pain of the pelvis and bladder) at age thirty. She had been sexually abused as a child. During her sexual abuse, she experienced both emotional pain and physical pain. She never told anyone about the abuse and she held all of that pain inside. She continued to re-experience that emotional pain over and over during her life. After twenty years, she finally developed physical pain. Although she received traditional treatment, she was not able to overcome her chronic pain until she was able to address the adversity and relieve herself of the burden she held inside for so many years.

There are two very important points to this story. First, at the time of her abuse, C. internalized all of her pain and emotions and held them inside, pretending they did not exist. Second, when C. experienced the abuse, she lost the ability to feel and process any other emotions or feelings. These are important aspects of maladaptive, or ineffective and inappropriate, coping that set the stage (in Hebb's terms, assembled cells in her brain) for the experience of future physical pain.

This is not C.'s fault; she was the victim here. (All too often we blame the victim for what happened and their "failure" to deal with the abuse.) First of all, the assault was not her fault. Second, her response of shutting down was the best coping mechanism she had at the time, and it allowed her to survive the abuse. Third, different people have different intrinsic abilities to cope and handle stressful experiences as well as different abilities to recover from stressful experiences. We call this capacity to handle stress *resilience*. At this point, we do not fully understand why some people seem to be born with more resilience than others, but this does seem to be the case. Severe trauma, such as torture, and regular, repeated stress can affect coping skills in anyone, no matter how much resilience they are born with. However, people do possess varying degrees of the resilience that helps them find support and develop the insight to process and overcome the effects of stress and the adverse experiences they have had in their lives.

Few people get through life without facing some significant adverse, stressful events. The potential to develop chronic pain is tied to the interaction between the number of stressful experiences (or adverse events) throughout a person's lifetime and that person's ability to cope and respond to these experiences. You will learn more about this in future chapters where I explore stress, adversity, suffering, and coping in greater depth.

The second part of my definition of chronic pain suggests that when a negative sensation has been internalized it is "holding one from being able to heal." This removes chronic pain from the realm of traditional medicine. Traditional medicine tends to view the body as a physical system with organs and organ systems that may go wrong and that may be repaired through using appropriate medications or surgical interventions. In many instances—such as a broken bone, hypertension, or infection—this may work very well, but with chronic pain as I have defined it, the disease is in the interaction of the brain, mind, and body and occurs, in part, because we may hold unresolved painful experiences within us. Therefore, successful treatment must address and relieve the underlying burden that holds us hostage to chronic pain. Until this is accomplished, one is essentially held captive by internalized pain that is not accessible to traditional methods that only treat the body.

My definition is also supported by our ability to interpret a sensation in our body as "pain" or as "not-pain." This last distinction is very important. It means that the neural pathways that experience pain have a parallel interpretation in the mind, and the interpretation of the pain sensation can lead to many different outcomes. Much depends on previous experience with pain and how those experiences were interpreted and internalized. It is important to understand this point as it is the foundation to the treatment activities provided in part 2 of this book.

When patients understand that the context for their interpretation of pain matters, they often realize that they were experiencing pain long before the onset of chronic physical pain. This new context also gives them a better understanding of how events that occurred earlier in their lives can contribute to their experience of physical pain. They begin seeing that we connect emotions and feelings with all types of pain and that, for the most part, those emotions are categorized in our mind as negative (fear, anger, anxiousness, sudden loss, humiliation, and so forth). Negative emotions are commonly experienced as *hurting inside,* which is another way of saying they are painful. This explains how physical pain *hurts* because of the emotional *and* cognitive (how we interpret pain in our mind) aspects associated with it. Although this concept may be difficult to understand on first reading, as we progress through this chapter and the rest of the book, these aspects of my definition of chronic pain will become increasingly clear.

Why Do We Have Pain?

Chronic pain—or lack of healing, as in my definition—is related to acute pain, but different. *Pain* is a sensation generated by a sensory event that has its origins somewhere in our bodily tissues. The sensation quickly travels to our brain to tell us that something is wrong. Generally, this is because we have had an injury or some type of tissue damage. We have very specific receptors in our skin, organs, bones, and most other tissues that help us feel pain. These receptors recognize the presence of painful (harmful) stimulation or damage and initiate the message that is sent to our brain. The message follows a very specific pathway that quickly moves from the tissues to the spinal cord to the brain to tell us that something is wrong: we have experienced damage to our body.

From acute pain to chronic pain

When we first experience pain it is *acute,* which means that it recently occurred. Acute pain happens to let us know that whatever we were doing (or whatever was happening to us) caused damage to our body. It tells us that we are in danger and should stop what we are doing and seek safety, help, possibly medical aid, and convalescence (or healing). After we do this, we should soon begin to heal, and the pain should decrease and generally disappear in a short amount of time relative to the severity of the damage and our basic state of health when healing begins. Generally, this process should be well under way in the first week after the injury and, depending on the severity of the damage, should be completed in no longer than a few months. With an injury or illness that causes acute pain, the sensation of pain serves a life-preserving function. In many instances it can save our lives. It is self-limiting and should generally have an endpoint when healing is complete.

In some instances, the pain continues and progresses for more than three months or beyond the normal period of healing. This is when the pain has become chronic. This process is not adaptive—that is, it does not help us do better in the world, it does not help us survive, and it does not help us learn. Rather, it can become overwhelmingly distracting and can have a dramatic, negative impact on our lives. Though chronic pain is common (as the statistics I reported earlier confirm), it is not *acceptable*. By this I mean it is not something we should be having, because it does not do us any good. Rather than serving a life-preserving function, it makes life worse.

When one has an acute injury and seeks help, the traditional medical model is to fix whatever injury has occurred. For example, if you slip and break your arm, the medical system will diagnose the break, reposition and cast the bone, and prescribe a medication to help relieve the pain involved. Generally, the sensation of pain with a broken bone is extraordinarily strong, negative, and consuming. It has the ability to take our attention away from any other thing we may be doing at the time of injury, but as was explained above, the pain itself should be time-limited. When this pain signal continues beyond a certain point after treatment of the injury, it becomes extremely distracting.

I noted earlier that when pain becomes chronic, doctors often use the same treatments that are used for acute pain, such as opioid medications, surgeries, injections, or implantable devices. For the most part, these treatments are at best partially successful for chronic pain. This mediocre success occurs for a number of reasons. First, the model does not always acknowledge the differences between acute pain and chronic pain, even though research done over the last twenty years has uncovered dramatic differences between acute and chronic pain. The most important difference, using my definition of chronic pain, is that when pain becomes chronic, it is a disease of the brain—that is, parts of the brain have changed the way they process information. Changes occur in the actual structure and function of the brain. Treatments used for acute pain arising from an illness or injury are not always effective for chronic pain and in many instances can actually increase the amount of pain a person experiences. This will be discussed more fully in chapter 6, which covers neuroplasticity.

Recent research has not been able to demonstrate that chronic pain always results from damage to the body nor has research found that this pain can be effectively treated with the same methods used to treat acute pain. For example, many people with osteoarthritis (damage to the joint) have no pain. Conversely, many people who *do* experience joint pain have X-rays of the joint that reveal no damage to that joint. The same is true of imaging done on the spine. Many people with evidence of damage to their spine experience no pain. Some have pain, yet there appears to be little relationship between the amount of damage in the spine, the frequency and intensity of the pain, and how much disability that pain causes. In the previous chapter, I related the story of a man I examined in the emergency room who had such dramatic degeneration of his cervical (neck) spine that it had impinged upon his spinal cord and, as a result, he could not move his upper and lower extremities. It was a medical emergency, and I had to quickly consult a neurosurgeon to surgically decompress his spine. When I asked the patient if he had ever experienced any neck pain, the answer was no. It was the most dramatic case of degeneration of the spine that I had ever seen with no evidence of pain.

For the most part, current medical practice only considers the probable area of damage that is causing the chronic pain and symptoms, and the results of diagnostic tests determine the treatment. Yet this approach often overlooks important aspects of how and why the patient experiences pain; it does not address the whole person.

> For example, when I first met with my patient "P.," a woman who had been involved in an industrial accident and had endured eight surgeries on her lumbar spine, she was experiencing symptoms of depression, had given up, and frankly wanted to die. She was scheduled to have one more surgery. Until we began working together, no one had asked her about

her past. No one bothered to find out about the abuse she had experienced as a teenager. No one took the time to ask how she handled her feelings when the abuse occurred or how she was handling her current feelings. P. had never realized that she had internalized the emotions associated with those past events. She did not even know she lacked the very learnable skills needed to process feelings in a healthy manner. Indeed, the only coping mechanism she had was to pretend that those feelings did not exist. Her coping method was to simply try to go on and be as strong as possible while ignoring any uncomfortable feelings that she was experiencing or had experienced in the past. This approach caused her to develop symptoms of depression and anxiety, the inability to sleep, and the expectancy that the future would be negative—all of which, as you will soon learn, are part of chronic pain.

P. was in a tremendous amount of physical pain, but she did not realize that her past emotional and social pain were connected to her present pain. In such a scenario, traditional medical treatments would not normally uncover the emotions associated with her past trauma and would fail to identify them as factors in her present chronic condition. Furthermore, even if these traditional medical providers had explored P.'s past and considered the nature of her coping skills as a factor in her treatment, most are not trained to help her apply them in addressing her chronic pain. With patients like P. who have psychiatric diagnoses and abuse issues, psychological counseling by people trained to deal with these specific problems is necessary.

What sets the stage for chronic pain?

Unlike P., most people who have an injury heal. Most people who have physical abnormalities such as osteoarthritis do not experience chronic pain. However, in some instances, as noted above, people do develop chronic pain. For example, only about 20 percent of people whose spinal discs are degenerating, or breaking down, will have chronic pain. Some of the research I have been involved in over the last ten years has examined the differences between people who go on to develop chronic pain and those who do not. I have already briefly discussed the results of this research and will provide further details later in this book. To summarize, people who are under a high degree of stress and have been under stress for a long time (possibly because of past adverse or traumatic events) are more likely to develop chronic pain. There are strong links between adverse experiences, the psychological and physical stress that results, and the development of chronic pain. Our research demonstrated that people with the conditions described below are also more likely to have chronic pain:

- *symptoms of depression*—feeling sad, a sense of worthlessness, a sense that your body no longer works, a sense that you can no longer do things you used to do, harsh self-judgment, and trying to change the past

- *catastrophic thinking processes*—expectations that things never go right and will always go wrong, dread of the future, and belief that things can only get worse

- *poor emotional self-care*—difficulty recognizing stress, poor coping, not recognizing emotions, the inability to process feelings and sensations inside of your body, and negative autobiographical narrative

If you reflect on the story of P., you will recognize that most of what we have described results from maladaptive thinking patterns. P. had clear symptoms of depression. She had a catastrophic view of the future. And no one had taught her the skills of self-care, how to deal with stress, or simply how to feel without fear. All of these maladaptive mechanisms will be explained in detail as we proceed through the book. It is important that you understand them and how they may contribute to your suffering. As you gain insight about these aspects of pain and suffering, you will be ready to learn the skills needed to relieve the burden that they impose on your life.

Traditional Treatment for Chronic Pain

Over the last twenty years, many studies have looked at how chronic pain affects the brain. With most diagnoses that involve pain, specific changes occur in the structure and function of the brain when the pain becomes

31

chronic. This means that chronic pain somehow changes the structure of nerve cells in the brain and negatively affects how those cells interact with one another and process information. This calls into question how we should treat chronic pain, because it appears that the most important organ affected is the brain. Why, then, would it make sense to simply try to stop the pain sensation using medications or to change the structure of the body part where the pain appears to be coming from unless there is evidence of direct impingement on nerves? These treatments often do not address the changes that have occurred in the brain of patients with chronic pain.

The mainstay of treatment for chronic pain has been opioid painkillers, such as Vicodin and OxyContin. They work on the part of the brain that turns the pain signal off. In clinical trials that have been ongoing for the past thirty years, opioids have been shown to reduce pain by approximately 20 to 30 percent when the pain is chronic. Unfortunately, this effect only lasts for about the first three months of use. Thereafter, opioids become progressively less effective and can actually begin to *increase* the experience of pain.

This occurs for a number of reasons. While a subset of patients with chronic pain do respond well to long-term opioid use, in most patients, the brain responds to opioids in a way that reduces the magnitude of their effect. Regular opioid use also changes the sites in their brain called *receptors* that the opioids interact with. The receptors become less abundant and less responsive to the opioids, a process called *down regulation*. Over time, this results in these patients becoming *tolerant* (less responsive) to the same dosage of medication. Then dosages must be increased, though an equivalent reduction in pain is seldom achieved. Moreover, the areas of the brain that are *antinociceptive*—that is, that reduce the pain signal— shut off and allow pain to continue unchecked throughout the brain. This phenomenon, called *hyperalgesia,* causes the patient's perception of pain to increase. Because the receptors that opioids interact with have so many different functions in the brain, patients also experience increased symptoms of depression, the inability to get restorative sleep, increased anxiety, less ability to experience joy, and dramatic changes in many hormones.

Probably the worst effect of long-term opioid use is addiction. This occurs because the brain becomes so accustomed to the opioids that it cannot function normally without them. The addicted person will go into painful withdrawal if the opioids are abruptly stopped. I will talk in more detail about this in the next chapter.

Many other medications are prescribed to the chronic pain patient, including nonsteroidal anti-inflammatory drugs (NSAIDs) and antiepileptic drugs such as Neurontin and Topamax, which can offer time-limited relief of symptoms but which seldom offer a permanent solution. Often chronic pain patients are given sedative hypnotics, the most common of which are benzodiazepines (such as Valium, Klonopin and Xanax) and sleeping aids (such as Ambien) along with opioids. These medications are also addictive, present a high risk of overdose, and can eventually create greater levels of depression, anxiety, and feelings of hopelessness. Other attempts to relieve symptoms for the chronic pain patient include injection of anti-inflammatory and numbing medication into the area assumed to be generating the pain. These treatments can offer temporary relief and, in rare cases, long-term relief. At still other times, implantable devices such as pumps that inject medication directly into the spine (*intrathecal* injections) are used to bring pain relief. These treatments can provide temporary relief, but if they include opioids they can lead to the same problems seen with oral opioid medications.

Various electrical and magnetic treatments have also been tried. *Spinal cord stimulation* has been a recent attempt to help with chronic pain. With this treatment, a device that creates an electrical signal is inserted into the back of the spinal column, providing a distraction to the pain sensation. This strategy appears to help specific types of pain but currently does not seem to offer a long-term remedy. *Transcranial magnetic stimulation* is an approach in which a magnetic pulse is applied to the brain in an attempt to disrupt the pain signal. This treatment appears to offer temporary relief in some pain syndromes. Other attempts have been made to apply electrical stimulation directly into the brain (deep brain stimulation). The results of these strategies have also been mixed, and the treatments are still being researched and refined.

Surgical interventions have been an important part of the treatment for chronic pain. In the United States we perform more surgeries of the spine than in any other country. All of the studies to date on surgical interventions of the spine show that while they may lead to structural improvement, they do not improve pain and functional status. As a rule, if the neurologic exam used in traditional medicine reveals abnormalities (muscle weakness, loss of sensation, or increase in reflexes), there is likely a problem with the spinal column or the nerves that exit it and surgery is deemed necessary. It is best if the least invasive procedure can be done. Unfortunately, the more invasive procedures change the anatomy of the spine and the surrounding muscles, and this in itself often leads to chronic pain. Replacing the discs of the spine is still in the experimental stage of development.

Total joint replacement surgeries have often been a blessing to patients with advanced degenerative joint disease. I have seen many patients come through the replacement surgery with complete resolution of pain. However, the lifesaving (or life-improving) procedure must be done with great precision in order to maintain the anatomy of the joint.

Many complementary treatments such as acupuncture, Qigong, osteopathic manipulation, chiropractic manipulation, yoga, and energy work, to mention a few, have shown good results for people with chronic pain. Most of these treatments attempt to tune in to the body's natural ability to heal. Many of these techniques are included in the multimodality treatments that we use at our treatment center and will be explained as the book progresses. Several of them, such as Qigong, a Chinese discipline that integrates physical postures, breathing techniques, mental focus, and other energy work, are key elements in the exercises found in part 2.

Often, the current treatments used for chronic pain offer temporary relief with questionable long-term outcomes and benefits. This may be due to the complexity of the changes that occur in the brain when pain becomes chronic.

A vicious cycle of negative experiences

Two of the worst outcomes that chronic pain has on the patient are (1) its effect on cognition (our ability to think and understand) and (2) its effect on emotions. Chronic pain produces a demonstrated reduction in the ability to think, to pursue a goal, and to regulate emotions. In order for the brain to return to balance and heal, we need to treat the diminished cognitive ability and the inability to regulate emotions.

For example, most chronic pain patients unintentionally create more pain by expecting that pain will always be present and that it will continue to worsen. This is referred to as *negative expectancy*. Negative expectancy creates anxiety, more pain, and more fear of pain. People with chronic pain, then, begin to live with the constant fear of more pain, and such negative thoughts and emotions only create the very increase in pain they fear.

Negative expectancy appears in other thinking patterns of chronic pain patients as well. For example, chronic pain patients often *ruminate,* which means they re-create the same thoughts again and again. Rumination that involves chronic pain generally has a negative narrative. This is especially true when one holds unresolved adverse feelings associated with negative past experiences. Rumination can create anxiety, worry, and the outlook of a negative future—that is, negative expectancy.

As chronic pain progresses, patients increasingly lose a sense of optimism, and this loss can also be thought of as negative expectancy. To be optimistic is to expect that a positive outcome will occur, and this has been shown to be the best form of coping. But people with chronic pain get to a point where they think they will always be in pain, as though they have been sentenced to a lifetime of pain. They lose hope for a positive future. This only serves to create more pain, as a lack of optimism is associated with poor coping skills.

Studies have shown that many chronic pain patients are under the impression that if they use or move their body, the pain will worsen. They falsely assume that any movement or activities, such as stretching, yoga, or tai chi and Qigong exercises, will make them feel pain, when in fact, such movements have been shown to help reduce the pain. They also falsely believe that they are unable to do much activity, and yet studies show that chronic pain patients are moving much more than they perceive themselves to be. In this way, an important element of chronic pain is the inability to recognize when movement is helpful or harmful.

These aspects of chronic pain reveal that chronic pain is a very complex disease and that most current treatments do not address the bulk of these complexities. It is not enough to simply focus on symptoms. We must address the underlying foundation that is holding the chronic pain patient hostage. Such an approach must address the cognitive, emotional, sensory, and spiritual aspects of chronic pain. Attempts to simply treat the assumed source of the pain most often fail because they do not address what has occurred in the brain as a result of the pain. The treatment of chronic pain must also consider that the brain is constantly changing and any stimulation that it receives can produce an effect. Therefore the successful treatment of chronic pain needs to address and change maladaptive thinking patterns and emotional processing while reducing stress, improving coping skills, and helping the patient learn to move in a pain-free manner.

Conclusion

The intent of this chapter was to help you understand that chronic pain is complex and that many people are affected by it. I hope you have learned that chronic pain is much more than just long-term physical pain. It is important to understand the new definition of chronic pain that I have proposed as *any sensation with a negative context in the mind that is holding one from being able to heal.* Therefore, experiencing anxiety, symptoms of depression, rejection, or the loss of a loved one is experiencing pain. This is true because all of these experiences create a negative feeling inside of us. Since this is the case and since all of these painful sensations are processed by the same neural networks in the brain, they can all set the groundwork for the future experience of pain by strengthening these networks. More important, they can keep us from healing.

It is also important to understand that there is not always a clear relationship between tissue damage and the source of pain when pain becomes chronic. This is supported by evidence that chronic pain is a disease of the brain. When this is understood it becomes clear that the brain must be treated in order to conquer chronic pain. This is why many traditional treatments have only been partially successful at best.

Finally, it is important to keep in mind that chronic pain is extraordinarily complex—it has a dramatic effect on cognition (thinking), perceptions, emotions, outlook, and hope. It can become totally consuming and change one's life in a very negative manner.

The mind and body have the ability to heal. My job and the job of this book will be to lead you on a path to balance and self-healing. In the next chapter, I will discuss the epidemic that has been created in our country by the prescribing of opioid painkillers. As you will see, this epidemic has had severe consequences. I will also explain the results of some recent research that compares chronic pain patients who are taking opioids with those who are not. You will gain a greater understanding of why we so urgently need non-opioid treatments for chronic pain.

. . .

3

Opioid Medications and Chronic Pain

Prescription opioids are overwhelmingly the most used treatment for acute and chronic pain. It is important that you, as a person who may suffer from chronic pain or may know someone who does, understand how opioid pain medications work and some of the problems that occur with their chronic use.

Over the last twenty years the use of opioid medications for chronic pain has skyrocketed. This has occurred despite the fact that there is little evidence that they are helpful and despite mounting evidence that they may be harmful. In this chapter, I will explain why this is the case and explore how the current epidemic of opioid use in our country came about. I will also explain the effects of opioids when they are taken for an extended period.

It is important to note that the body is equipped with a mechanism to produce its own opioids. Therefore, opioids are part of the brain's natural environment and are involved in many natural processes that help us adapt to the conditions of our ever-changing environment. These natural substances are important in our body; when we introduce additional opioids, normal body processes can be disrupted as the receptors for our naturally occurring opioids, such as endorphins, are hijacked. So, if you are prescribed opioid pain medications (or know someone who is), you should know all of their potential effects. These effects go far beyond the original intent of reducing pain.

But first, let's look at some simple definitions. As background, it is important to recognize that the prototype of all opioids is morphine.

Morphine is a naturally occurring substance that is similar to—and is derived from—the opium resin that is extracted from certain types of poppy plants. (There are more than two hundred varieties of poppy, but only four are known to produce opium resin.)

- An *opioid* is any chemical structure that resembles the structure of morphine and has a similar pharmacologic effect.
- An *opiate* is any of the naturally occurring alkaloid resins found in the opium poppy (papaver somniferum). Morphine and codeine are examples.

Opioids and Their Effects

The opioids most people think of are taken externally (called *exogenous* opioids). Examples of these are morphine, heroin, and oxycodone. As noted earlier, the body also naturally produces opioids (known as *endogenous* opioids). They serve many important roles in the body, and most of these roles will be reviewed below. The naturally occurring opioids that are produced in the body are endorphins, enkephalins, dysnorphins, and endomorphins.

Opioids are among the oldest known drugs, and their use is thought to predate any recorded medical history. Opioids are best known for their effect on pain. They have been shown to work quite well on acute pain, end-of-life pain, and cancer pain. Interestingly, opioids do not stop pain, but instead they change the perception of pain. The effect is simply to dull our attention to pain. People report that the pain is still there but that it no longer matters. Altogether, opioids decrease the ability to perceive pain, change the interpretation of it, and change the emotional reaction to pain. In fact, multiple studies have shown that low doses of opioids that are not able to affect physical pain *can* have an effect on the emotional reaction to pain. Thus, the first level of pain that opioids can affect is the emotional interpretation of pain. (Remember, although the brain processes all types of pain in a similar manner, the mind interprets pain in many different ways.)

Opioids also produce the experience of euphoria. *Euphoria* is an intense state or feeling of pleasure, happiness, and well-being. This mental state can occur naturally or can be induced by drugs. The euphorigenic (tending to cause euphoria) effect produced by opioids is probably the most dangerous aspect of this drug class and helps explain why people seek them out for recreational use, which can lead to addiction. However, as we will see, this effect is time-limited—that is, the effect of killing pain and the euphoric effect decrease over time when the drug is used repeatedly. This is where most of the trouble and misunderstanding about the use of these medications occurs.

Opioid receptors

A *receptor* is a structural unit in a cell membrane. Its function is to interact with a chemical, such as an opioid or a neurotransmitter (brain chemicals that carry signals from one brain cell neuron to another), and cause a reaction to occur. We have many kinds of receptors, and they are critical for transmitting information throughout the brain and nervous system. There are four known opioid receptors.

Opioid receptors were first proposed to exist in 1954 by Arnold H. Beckett and Alan F. Casy, reported in the journal *Nature* and again in the *Journal of Pharmacology*. But it was not until 1973 that researchers were first able to produce evidence of their existence. In that year, Johns Hopkins School of Medicine researchers Candace Pert and Solomon Snyder were able to show that opioids bind to specific areas in the brain. (The researchers made this discovery by using opioids that were labeled with radioactive material that enabled the opioids to be examined in the brain.) Over the last few decades, four opioid receptors have been identified. Named *mu, kappa, delta,* and *nociceptin/orphanin,* these opioid receptors are found throughout the central and peripheral nervous systems. They can be activated by either exogenous or endogenous opioids. They have a wide range of effects that include the ability to reduce pain.

Once opioids interact with opioid receptors, a series of chemical reactions occur inside the nerve cell that produce both physiological and psychological effects. These effects can be experienced as both minor and dramatic changes of mood across a range of feelings, such as the following:

- the satisfaction of attaining a certain social status or career success
- the enjoyment of food

THE CHEMICAL REACTIONS BEHIND PAIN SIGNALS

When opioids interact with opioid receptors, a series of chemical reactions occur inside the nerve cell. This chain of reactions is referred to as the *G protein signaling pathway*. This is one of the many second messenger systems that acts in the body. *Second messenger systems* are molecules that relay signals from receptors on the cell surface to target molecules inside the cell. They are attached to the receptor and become active when the receptor becomes active. It is almost as if there were a series of chemicals attached to the inside of the receptor. As soon as a substance interacts with the receptor, the series of chemicals that are attached to the receptor become active. Once this occurs, an effect is seen inside the cell.

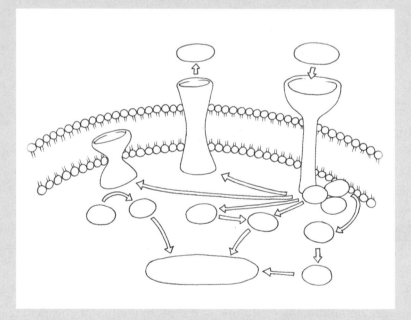

Figure 1. The three cuplike figures within the cell membrane represent mu opioid receptors, two of which are about to interact with an opioid outside of the cell membrane. The circles and arrows inside of the cell represent the G protein second messenger system that becomes active when an opioid interacts with the mu receptor system.

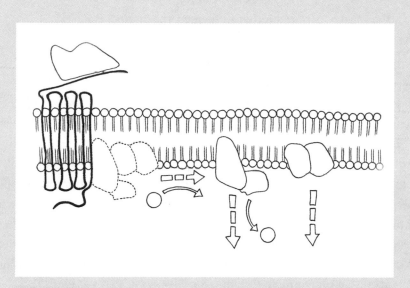

Figure 2. Here is a more detailed view of the system. On the left, spanning the cell membrane, is the receptor. The shapes within the cell membrane and inside the cell between the arrows are the components of the second messenger system that come together and become active when a substance such as an opioid interacts with the receptor. This second messenger system is the G protein system that is related to the mu opioid receptor.

When the G protein signaling pathway is activated by an opioid, a channel opens that enables the nerve cell to change the electrical signal that it carries, making it more difficult for the nerve cells to deliver the message of pain. The psychological effect is a reduction in perceived pain. Opioids can also inhibit the release of certain neurotransmitters that are important in the transmission of pain. Thus, opioid receptors can reduce the perception of pain in multiple ways. Try to recall a time when you were in pain but suddenly became distracted by intense joy or deep involvement in some activity. Many people report that pain seems to disappear during such episodes. This may well be an effect of internally produced opioids.

- the comfort produced by meaningful social interaction
- the sensual attraction that influences the choice of a sexual partner

Important to our discussion, these effects also include changing the perception of pain. *(See diagrams on pages 42 and 43.)*

Besides the ability of opioids to change the perception of pain, they are involved in many other important brain functions.

For example, opioids and their receptors play a key role in our ability to move. We also know that abnormal opiate transmission is involved in a number of diseases and has even been linked to eating disorders—people with these disorders appear to receive an abnormal amount of enjoyment (thought to result from reduced amounts of natural opioids and their receptors) from obtaining and consuming food. Opioids also produce changes in endocrine function, in the function of the gut, in the cardiac system, and in the immune system.

Opioid receptors are probably best known for their role in mood regulation. Interestingly, people with depression have alterations in the availability of opioid receptors. When these opioid receptors do not function properly and when there is a decreased number of functional receptors, a depressive-like state occurs. If this situation is prolonged, a state of depression occurs. One interesting study found that when patients with major depressive disorder experienced a state of sadness, there was a dramatic decrease in available opioid receptor binding as compared to a group of people who were healthy.

Since opioid pain medications affect mood, it is not unusual for chronic pain patients who are on long-term use of opioid painkillers to have symptoms of depression—these symptoms may be the result of being on the opioid painkillers and the associated changes in the receptors that occur after prolonged use. This is why antidepressants are seldom effective in chronic pain patients. If one does not have a normal *mu receptor system* intact, it is impossible for antidepressant medications to have a positive effect on mood. Further, it is not unusual for chronic pain patients who are on opioid painkillers to detach from social situations and isolate themselves from other people. This, too, results from the changes that occur in the mu receptor system after prolonged use.

Most of the patients I see who have been on prolonged opioid pain medication for chronic pain do not have the ability to experience joy. The part of the brain that would normally tell them that they like something and that it feels good has been significantly altered by the extended use of opioid painkillers—so they simply cannot experience positive emotions. This only exacerbates perceived pain.

OPIOID RECEPTORS AND ADDICTION

Mu opioid receptors have been implicated in the reinforcing effects of opioid drugs that lead to addiction. The transition from the first use of opioids to addiction involves dramatic structural and functional changes in the brain's mu opioid receptor system. Interestingly, the *kappa opioid receptor* is involved in the dysphoria that accompanies the withdrawal process that occurs when opioids are abruptly stopped after prolonged use. This receptor system contributes to the dysphoric mood state (feelings of irritability and dissatisfaction) that often occurs in mood disorders and often for an extended period of time after patients have stopped taking opioids. It is important for someone coming off prolonged use of opioids to be under the care of a professional trained in dealing with the potential complications.

We can see that opioids and their four receptor types in the brain are involved in multiple functions. Most of these functions are extremely important to our well-being and enable us to adapt to our environment. Although doctors may prescribe opioids as a treatment for pain, they rarely provide patients with this level of information about how opioids may affect multiple aspects of normal brain function. As a result, most patients are not aware that the psychological manifestations of these changes can be dramatic. As will be discussed extensively in chapter 6, most chronic pain patients who take opioid pain medications for long periods of time experience extensive changes in the brain, most of which become maladaptive and do not serve them. This is why I believe that when patients are given opioids for chronic pain, they need to understand that using these medications can negatively alter multiple functions that our naturally produced opioids are responsible for and that, without treatment, these alterations can be prolonged. This is also why it is important that we develop alternative treatments for chronic pain instead of relying on opioids.

Opioid Prescribing Practices in the United States

Opioids, as noted, have been used both medically and recreationally for thousands of years. In the United States, the nonmedical use of opioids was made a criminal act in 1914 by the Harrison Narcotics Tax Act. This act was strictly enforced until the 1990s, when the use of opioids was restricted to the treatment of acute pain, cancer pain, and end-of-life care. Among the medical community and legislators, there had been a fear that the long-term use of opioids for chronic noncancer pain would lead to addiction and that chronic pain would eventually become unresponsive to opioids. In the 1990s it was recognized that a large portion of Americans suffered from chronic noncancer pain and that these people were not being adequately treated. At about that time a series of events occurred that led to the liberal prescribing of opioids for moderate to severe chronic noncancer pain. What follows is a brief overview of this changed practice and how the change has contributed to a general overprescribing of opioids, which is currently at epidemic levels.

In the late 1980s many doctors began to question the assumption that the use of chronic opioids would lead to addiction. At about this time pharmaceutical companies began a vigorous campaign endorsing the use of opioids for chronic noncancer pain. In the 1990s a letter appeared in the *New England Journal of Medicine* that reported the results of an observational study on about 12,000 patients who had been prescribed chronic opioid therapy. This letter reported that very few of these patients went on to develop addiction. Soon after, the journal *Pain* reported on another observational study that found positive results with little aberrant behavior when a modest number of patients were prescribed long-term opioid therapy for chronic noncancer pain. (However, this study involved only twenty-four patients. Two of them, or about 8 percent, reported aberrant behavior during the opioid therapy.)

During this same period, a number of physicians were being sued for not adequately treating pain, and the American Pain Society, to which I belong, pronounced pain to be the fifth vital sign. (A *vital sign* is a body function considered by health care providers as a key indicator of physiological state. The four other vital signs are heart rate, temperature, respiration rate, and blood pressure.) Slowly, at first, and then progressively faster, the practice of prescribing opioids for chronic noncancer pain became commonplace.

Along with the increased practice of prescribing opioids, the rate of overdose deaths involving opioid pain medications began to rise. In 1995 this increase became noticeable. At the same time, clinical trials that examined the use of opioids for chronic noncancer pain were ongoing. Interestingly, the results of these studies were disappointing. Overall, there is about a 30 percent decrease in pain for the first three months (or less) reported in these trials. None of these studies examined quality of life or improvement of function. All of these studies excluded anyone who had extensive medical or psychiatric issues in addition to chronic pain. In other words, all patients with depression, addiction, or any other psychiatric issues were excluded from the studies. Despite this very tightly chosen subject pool, the results were *still* overwhelmingly disappointing. That is, even among people with no other complaint but pain who were relatively healthy, the use of opioids for chronic pain did not produce significant and lasting results. Over 50 percent of subjects dropped out because of inadequate pain control, adverse side effects, misuse, or a combination of these problems. In three longer-term, eighteen-month observation studies only 14 percent of subjects were still using the medication by the end of the study. Only an estimated one out of thirty-five patients was helped by prolonged opioid therapy, and there was evidence of worse quality of life and functioning.

Despite these findings, many health care providers (and most patients) had believed that chronic opioid therapy could help patients with chronic pain. This misperception is still prevalent in the medical community today, and I do not know how to explain it. I do not think my colleagues are trying to do harm. It is easy to understand the moral argument that patients with chronic pain should be treated in some way to reduce their suffering. No one wants to see people suffer! But the evidence from clinical attempts to prove that opioids are helpful is poor. This makes it difficult to understand why this perception continues. It also seems clear that the practice of prescribing opioids has contributed to an epidemic of overuse and overdose.

Many of my physician colleagues are at a loss about how to treat the vast number of patients they see who have chronic pain. In the primary care setting, as many as 60 percent of patients have complaints involving chronic pain. I know that at this point many physicians feel hopeless in attempting to treat chronic pain. This is understandable. Even with the evidence that opioid painkillers seem to do more harm than good with chronic pain, many physicians, perhaps because of the success of these drugs with acute pain and even with some chronic pain patients, continue to prescribe them. They want to alleviate their patients' suffering, and many simply do not have an alternative plan for addressing the epidemic level of chronic pain in the United States.

Since 1999 there has been a 300 percent increase in the sale of opioid painkillers. Opioids cause more overdose deaths than all other medications combined. According to the Centers for Disease Control and Prevention, as of 2011, each day more than forty people die from overusing prescription painkillers. In 2008, these prescription drugs were involved in 14,800 overdose deaths. This is more than the *combined* deaths resulting from the better-known "street drugs" cocaine and heroin. In 2011, there were 420,040 visits to the emergency room that were related to the nonmedical use of opioid painkillers. This cost society an estimated $55.7 billion in the year 2007 alone. These statistics are staggering and point to the epidemic that has occurred, for the most part, as a result of prescribing practices of opioid pain medications in the United States.

The use of the medications Vicodin and Norco (which consist of a combination of the opioid hydrocodone and acetaminophen) in the United States accounts for almost 100 percent of the use of these medications worldwide. That is to say, we consume the vast majority of these medications in the U.S. Clearly there is no explanation for this statistic, as epidemiological studies of pain show equal amounts of pain in countries worldwide. Additionally, in the United States we consume 80 percent of the world supply of another opioid, oxycodone. Again, this statistic appears to have no logical explanation.

Epidemiological studies have shown that women are much more likely to have chronic pain than men. Of all Americans with chronic pain about 65 percent are women, and there are certain pain diagnoses, such as fibromyalgia and irritable bowel syndrome (IBS), where overwhelmingly, women are principally affected (fibromyalgia, 93 percent; IBS, 65 percent). An equally troubling finding is that there is a dramatic increase in women experiencing opioid painkiller overdoses. The CDC reported in 2010 approximately eighteen women died every day from opioid painkiller overdose, which accounted for 6,600 deaths in that year. The number of women who died per year from opioid prescription overdose increased five-fold from 1999 to 2010.

In 2012 health care providers wrote 259 million prescriptions for opioid painkillers in the United States. That is more than enough for each adult in the country to have a prescription for painkillers. In many states there are more prescriptions for opioid painkillers written than there are residents!

Recently, the Food and Drug Administration (FDA) approved the use of two powerful, purely hydrocodone pain medications. This occurred even though an FDA committee panel voted 11 to 2 against the approval and a committee recommended not to approve one of the medications.

Studies such as those cited above are not always easy to understand, but it should be clear that they do not support the use of opioids for chronic pain on many fronts. It should also be clear by now that I believe that we lack any good evidence that opioid pain medications are the right answer for chronic pain (although there appears to be a very small subset of chronic pain patients who may benefit from opioid therapy). As can be seen from the statistics, the cost of opioid medications dramatically outweighs the benefit, and if indeed chronic pain is a disease of the brain, we are missing the point by treating it with opioids. Statistics such as these should be taken seriously by both health care workers and legislators. They motivate me to continue my work toward nondrug treatment of chronic pain.

Our Study of Chronic Pain Patients

Multiple studies have shown that chronic pain patients in the United States are not doing well despite multiple attempts at adequate treatment. The patients who are in long-term opioid therapy have a number of factors in common. These include symptoms of depression, a history of adversity (negative and stressful events), physical inactivity, obesity, poor physical and mental health, and multiple areas of pain.

To assess the current state of chronic pain in the United States, my colleagues and I at the Hazelden Betty Ford Foundation and Loma Linda University School of Medicine conducted an online survey of 1,009 people who had chronic pain. We wanted to gain an understanding of how frequently they experienced pain, how long it lasted, and how severe the pain was. We also wanted to get a sense of the respondents' quality of life and how pain had affected their lives, how much adversity they had experienced, their use of medications, their perception of dependence, their satisfaction with their current treatment, and whether they had or feared dependency.

The survey was conducted from June to July, 2014. The results were statistically valid with a 3 percent margin of error. Essentially, this means that our results can be generalized across the entire adult population of people with chronic pain in the United States. When these studies are analyzed we calculate the number of subjects who responded as a percentage of the total population. Thus, if 50 percent of the subjects responded to a question positively, a 3 percent margin of error tells us that 47 to 53 percent of the overall target population would have a positive response.

It was not surprising that the major cause of pain in our subjects was lower back pain, followed by headache, neck pain, osteoarthritis, and fibromyalgia. Back pain and work-related injuries were more prevalent in men than women, whereas headaches, fibromyalgia, irritable bowel syndrome, and abdominal pain were more prevalent in women. The most dramatic finding was that over 97 percent of the respondents reported that they had experienced unresolved traumatic events, such as physical, emotional, or sexual abuse or unresolved grief over the loss of a loved one earlier in life.

I have already noted a study I conducted with my colleagues in 2008, where we asked chronic pain patients how many thought that death would be a better alternative to their current state and half said that it would be, but after six months of opioid therapy the percentage *increased* to 68 percent. Clearly, opioids produced a negative effect on outlook and hope that led to thoughts of death. We have to ask if a given therapy is actually effective when it appears to be associated with increased thoughts of suicide.

In the 2014 survey, the most commonly prescribed medications were opioids. Almost half (48 percent) of the respondents were prescribed three or more medications for pain. More than one out of three respondents (35 percent) stated that they had drug dependence related to their treatment. One out of twenty (5 percent) reported using illegal drugs, while one out of four patients (24 percent) had used more medication than they had been prescribed, and 24 percent had fears of becoming dependent on their medications. All patients stated that chronic pain had a dramatic effect on their lives, but many more of the patients on opioids stated that chronic pain had a significant negative effect on their lives.

We compared responses from those taking opioids with those who were not. Opioid users reported worse quality of life, higher levels of pain, worse functional status, and more symptoms of depression. Other studies have shown the same results. These findings support my observations of the patients I see. Moreover, when these patients are taken off of opioids and given adequate non-opioid treatment, they dramatically improve.

Results from our 2014 study not only show the effect that chronic pain has on those who suffer from it in the United States, they also suggest that many of the current treatments that are medication-based are inadequate. An encouraging finding from the survey was that 89 percent of respondents were not satisfied with using medications as the sole form of their treatment, and 80 percent stated that if an alternative treatment were available, they would be willing to reduce or stop the medications they take.

I find this last result extremely encouraging. It tells me that most patients with chronic pain in this country are open to and would seek alternatives to medication.

Conclusion

In this chapter, we have learned the basic way that opioids work and all the effects that opioids have on the brain and behavior. We have also seen that the current prescribing practices of opioids in the United States markedly increased in the 1990s, leading to significant negative consequences. This prescribing trend occurred despite multiple studies that have shown that opioid pain medications have not proven to be helpful when used long-term for the treatment of chronic pain. I also shared the results of an online survey that my colleagues and I completed that confirms that chronic pain patients continue to suffer despite opioid- and other medication-based treatment. However, it is encouraging to know that almost all patients want an alternative to the current treatment and would be willing to stop or at least reduce medications if such a treatment were available. In part 2, I will present some drug-free techniques that show promise. But before we get there, you need to know more about your own brain.

In the next chapter, I will explain how your brain is organized and how it works. It is important that you understand this because, as mentioned previously, chronic pain is a disease of the brain. The brain is a complex organ with the magnificent power to "reprogram" itself, which is essential in treating this disease. Understanding this capacity is an important step in reducing the negative experience of chronic pain.

• • •

4

Do Addiction and Chronic Pain Have Similarities?

During my career I have seen many interesting patients, some with just chronic pain or addiction and some with both. I have consistently observed similarities between patients with chronic pain and those with addiction, but until recently my observations had no scientific basis. Previous studies had examined areas of the brain involved in disease processes such as depression and anxiety, but only recently have studies examined chronic pain and addiction. These studies have found evidence suggesting that there is a great deal of overlap in the areas of the brain involved in addiction and in chronic pain. These brain areas are part of networks of nerve cells that enable one to process negative emotions, pay attention to internal states, and attend to what is needed to accomplish goal-directed tasks. In this chapter, you will learn that in both chronic pain and addiction, these areas do not function in a normal fashion.

Many of you may wonder why we would explore the question of whether there are similarities in the disease process of chronic pain and that of addiction. First, since both processes affect the same brain areas, our ongoing studies have shown that some of the treatments explained in this book appear to be successful with both diseases. This is important because we have a much longer and more successful record with nondrug methods of treating addiction than we do with nondrug methods of treating chronic pain. Second, as noted, there is a substantial overlap among people with addiction and people with chronic pain. We have seen many people misuse drugs in part as a way to deal with chronic pain. If this has been your experience, you will have a personal interest in the similarities of these diseases. And third, finding this overlap is new and unexpected, and breakthroughs like this are always exciting in that they can open the door to new treatment approaches.

I have taken the liberty of expanding on basic recent research that has been done on the brains of patients with *both* chronic pain and addiction to fine-tune the treatment I use for just chronic pain. When you understand what these studies mean in practical terms, you will find it easier to understand how and why they apply to treating the complex problem of chronic pain. Working with people who have both diseases has helped me see the similarities between the two diseases not in terms of symptoms, like "how much it hurts" or "the quality of the pain," but in terms of *how these diseases have affected the ways people think, process emotions, and lose hope.* I have been amazed by the similarities I see between these separate disease processes.

Chronic Pain and Addiction

Addiction is recognized as a chronic, relapsing disease that involves the constant need to attain addictive substances, loss of control over their intake, harmful and illegal behaviors, and negative emotional states including anxiety and depressed mood. There is a withdrawal state that occurs when access to the drug is not possible. It is as though the addict has been taken over by the substance so much that it rules her life. This state of constant concern over either obtaining the drug, using it, recovering from its effects, or dealing with its withdrawal is characterized by rumination—the drug is almost the only thing the addict thinks about. At this point, life becomes increasingly difficult, and the addict gradually loses the capacity to experience pleasure and joy in life.

Recall that in chapter 2, I defined chronic pain as "any sensation with a negative context in the mind that is holding one from being able to heal." The constant, relentless sensation of pain leads one to continually focus on pain and the negative emotional states and ongoing attempts to escape from these states. As the disease progresses, life itself becomes more and more painful, and there is less and less ability to experience pleasure and joy.

As you think about these definitions of addiction and chronic pain, you can see many similarities. In both cases, as the disease progresses it becomes increasingly painful to the individual. This pain can be both physical and emotional. The negative emotional states that occur with constant substance use and the withdrawal that follows are similar to the emotional states that people with chronic pain experience. Both diseases place the person in a nearly steady state of negative emotions (though the ups and downs may seem like a roller coaster to those around the patient). Both diseases are not only physically and emotionally painful; they also cause a kind of social pain by the isolation the person typically experiences. And both motivate those who suffer from them to attempt to escape from the pain. For the most part, these attempts are not successful and only lead to more pain.

It is not surprising that many people with addiction go on to develop chronic pain *or* had preexisting chronic pain that served as an entry point to the cycle of addictive use and withdrawal.

Shared predisposing factors

The similarities of addiction and chronic pain go beyond the characteristics of the disease states. We have learned that the diseases also share some of the same *predisposing factors*—that is, conditions that increase the likelihood a person might develop chronic pain or addiction. In earlier chapters, we have seen that many patients with chronic pain have a history of stressful events that have predisposed them to the later development of chronic pain. I have given examples of patients I have seen who had early childhood adversity and were not able to adequately cope with that stress and, consequently, are under a high degree of chronic stress. In chapter 2, I explained how previous pain experience affects the areas of the brain that process pain and that, as this experience is repeated, these areas are strengthened—they lower the threshold to send messages of pain—in a process called cell assembly. This sets the stage for future pain experience, especially if these early pain experiences were not adequately coped with and the burden they caused was not relieved. This happens when we do not process the emotional pain or effectively deal with the physical pain and instead hold the feeling internally, ignoring it, trying to forget it, or trying to cover it up with other activities. For people with this experience, it is often just a matter of time until they develop chronic pain. Thus, if you have a history of painful experiences, and if you also do not deal with those painful experiences successfully, you have prepared the brain for repeated negative emotional states. Moreover, frequently repeating or reliving painful emotional states can cause more and more pain. This can be experienced as a mental/emotional event or it may have a physical component, or both.

I believe that people who go from a state of experimental, social, or recreational drug use to constant use are most likely treating internal pain. Many of my patients have told me that the first time they took a substance like alcohol, cocaine, or an opioid painkiller, they found relief from the internal unease or negative emotional state that had plagued them for as long as they could remember. Many of these people also describe chronic symptoms of depression or other negative internal states that were relieved by that substance. Though such pain is not the same as the physical pain we associate with arthritis or other medical conditions, remember that in the brain, pain is pain. I believe that the euphoric state associated with drug use stops people from experiencing some negative internal states and that these states are pain. Let's explore these negative emotional states.

Negative Emotional States

Negative emotional states are a part of life. All of us can remember periods of life when we experienced particularly painful situations that led to negative emotional states. For the most part, we have been able to adequately cope with these emotions and return to a state of relative balance. For some people, however, these emotions become overwhelming and cannot be adequately processed, so they are not able to handle the onslaught of emotional pain. Recent studies have shown that the inability to handle negative emotional states appropriately often marks the beginning of the diseases of chronic pain and addiction.

Specific networks in the brain are involved in processing emotions. In certain instances, these networks malfunction and cannot adequately process emotions. This usually occurs during periods of high stress, such as when one has had an acute injury that causes intense pain or when one is beginning to use substances to cope with the stressors of life. I have treated many patients who, during very stressful experiences in their lives, either developed pain or began to use substances in an addictive manner. The studies mentioned above suggest that this occurs because the brain networks that handle negative emotions become overwhelmed and constantly experiencing unresolved negative emotions creates internal states of pain. As the brain processes these painful internal states, the part of the brain that enables us to value and enjoy a positive experience (in essence, "rewards" us with pleasurable feelings) is overwhelmed with negative feelings (a kind of "anti-reward"). This creates the opportunity for chronic pain and addiction to begin. As we will discuss in the sections on treating chronic pain, being able to identify these negative emotional states and to properly process them—including developing the ability to determine when and why they started—is an important component of my approach to the treatment for pain.

Many studies have examined predisposing factors to the development of both chronic pain and addiction. They found that patients who went on to develop persistent pain had symptoms of depression, anxiety, a negative mindset related to past adverse events, and the inability to handle past and present stress. Thus, if you have had a number of negative experiences in life that have become a part of your personal narrative, and/or you are under a tremendous amount of stress, you may come to expect that outcomes will always be negative, and this can lead to the overwhelming negative emotional states that often trigger both persistent pain and addiction.

When my colleagues and I interviewed patients who developed chronic pain and addiction, we found that most of them had used alcohol or other drugs to treat negative emotional states even before they developed physical pain. Almost all of them (97 percent) stated that they had experienced an adverse event (such as abuse or the loss of a loved one) prior to the development of chronic pain or addiction. In other studies we have looked at involving patients with just chronic pain, over 90 percent of these people reported unresolved feelings over adverse events in their past. Thus, we concluded that experiencing highly stressful events that result in persistent negative emotional states, such as abuse or other trauma, is a predisposing factor for changes in important areas of the brain that contributes to both chronic pain and addiction.

Default mode network

The brain is able to focus on certain tasks by disengaging from other tasks. For example, as you began reading this book you shifted your attention away from other tasks and internal experiences and put it on the task of reading, which involves comprehending the words, sentences, paragraphs, and chapters. As you do so, you understand the story the book tells about the nature of chronic pain and hopefully also connect it to your life. If you then stop for a moment and focus your attention inward to ask yourself questions, such as why you are reading this book and how the ideas it presents apply to your life, you are in a "task-negative" state. This is simply the act of taking attention away from an outside stimuli (the words on the page) or task (reading a book) and putting that attention inward (processing the myriad thoughts and feelings that the ideas in the book elicit), thereby disengaging from the specific task of reading the book. The neural network that allows one to achieve a task-negative state was first described by researcher Marcus Raiche in 2001 as the *default mode network*. This shift in the brain is comparable to moving from an active processing mode on a computer to a resting mode or default mode. At any time you should be able to switch from a state that is trying to accomplish a specific task to a task-negative state.

Recent research has shown that people with both chronic pain and addiction have problems achieving task-negative states (default mode). This is probably because the story or narrative in their head is extremely negative and the sensation of pain that accompanies both diseases dominates their thought processes. This negative narrative captures their attention, and they are engrossed in negative thought patterns accompanied by strong negative emotions. In the example above, instead of being able to achieve the task-negative state of objectively processing your thoughts and feelings about what you have been reading, your attention might be diverted by the emotional and/or physical pain that defines the negative narrative of the life story you carry—often rooted in adverse experiences from your past—preventing you from taking full advantage of any helpful advice this or any book might offer. Similar patterns have been found for people who are chronically depressed, who are anxious, or who have experienced traumatic events. As was discussed in chapter 2, when you ruminate on negative thoughts (common with both chronic pain and addiction), you are not able to switch into a contemplative mode.

When a person is caught up in negative thoughts and pain and unable to disengage from that narrative and achieve a default mode of effectively disengaging from the narrative, that person views the world from a negative perspective. This is an important aspect of chronic pain and it is also true of addiction. As you discover more about the brain and mind in later chapters and begin the exercises in the second part of this book, it will be important that you learn to go into the default mode and practice achieving a quiet mind. This will allow you to disengage from the sensation of pain.

Goal-directed thought

Specific areas of the brain are responsible for taking attention and focusing it on those aspects of the environment that allow us to accomplish goal-directed tasks. This capacity allows us to make our way through life more efficiently. Without this ability, life becomes difficult and highly stressful. Studies have shown that in both chronic pain and addiction, the areas of the brain that keep a person's attention on task, select which aspects of the environment to pay attention to, and prevent negative emotions from being a distraction are not adequately functioning. These diseases also diminish the capacity to recognize when a goal-directed task is failing. This is why people with chronic pain and addiction have trouble staying focused on tasks and completing goal-directed behavior.

Those of you who experience chronic pain are well aware of how distracting the pain can be and know that it often takes you away from completing tasks. If this happens often enough, you may even begin to think that you lack the ability to accomplish anything. As chronic pain progresses, this problem increases. In chapter 2, we described an extreme example of this distorted thinking pattern that occurs in some chronic pain patients where they are not able to accurately perceive their movements and even come to think that they are unable to move. People with addiction experience similar distortions in their thinking. Their attention is dominated by their attempts to acquire and take mood-altering substances, replacing more productive goal-directed behavior. Just as chronic pain (and the fear of pain) preoccupies the pain patient, drug acquisition and use preoccupies the addict's thinking. For those with chronic pain, addiction, or both, adaptive goal-directed behavior is difficult to accomplish.

Internal surveillance

Just as your brain has the ability to focus your attention on the external environment, it also has the ability to focus on the internal environment, a state called *internal surveillance*. As you are reading this book, for example, you are using your eyes to see the words and you are putting letters into words and words into sentences in order to comprehend what the book is trying to convey. If you stop reading for a second and put your attention inside of your body, you can simply perceive how it feels. You may learn, for example, that you feel hungry, calm, anxious, or something else you cannot name. Although anyone can do internal surveillance at any time, this ability has been dramatically diminished for people with chronic pain and addiction. All of the attention placed inside of their body becomes focused on negative internal cues that tell them they are not well and pain predominates. They lose the ability to survey their internal state without making a negative judgment. You will read more about this aspect of chronic pain as you go through the book, and I will present treatment strategies that allow you to do internal surveillance without this kind of harsh negative judgment.

Conclusion

While chronic pain and addiction are very different disease processes, we have learned that they have many things in common. We have seen that similar areas of the brain are involved in both diseases, and this means that many of the symptoms and behaviors are similar as well. This discovery has set the stage for developing a new approach to treating both diseases and has led to encouraging research findings, new approaches to research, and continued advances in treatment.

It is not uncommon for both people with chronic pain and people with addiction to feel that their lives are out of control and that they can no longer determine the direction their lives are going because factors outside of their control have taken over. We have explored how negative emotional states predominate in people with chronic pain or addiction so that they are unable to accomplish goal-directed behavior or achieve a task-negative state. We have shown how they can also have their attention fixed on the constant uncomfortable feelings that are part of their ongoing internal state. This is a very uncomfortable situation that creates considerable suffering. In the next chapter, you will learn some important information about the human brain and how it works. After a brief introduction of some general principles about the brain, I will focus on those areas of the brain that are affected by chronic pain.

. . .

5

The Brain

It is a huge challenge to try to incorporate all that is important about an organ as complex as the brain in one chapter. For our purposes, I have limited the information to critical, specific aspects of the brain that reveal how the brain becomes altered with chronic pain. I will also describe the basic physical principles of how neurons (nerve cells) work. I will explain why the brain should be viewed as an *information processing system* and how we are far from understanding how that processing works, especially when it comes to the creation of *consciousness,* which, as you will see, is important to understanding how we process pain. Don't worry if you do not remember all the technical terms or the structure of the brain. What is important is that you get a general idea about how the different brain functions contribute to how we experience chronic pain and how we can eventually change the experience for the better.

I will begin with a brief history of the search for the seat of consciousness. Next, I will describe the neuron and then talk about how groups of neurons come together as functional units to create mental activity. I will then discuss how the information processing activities of the brain can become altered by chronic pain. The chapter will close with a brief discussion of specific areas of the brain that are changed by chronic pain.

Much of this chapter will focus on the *cortex*. The cortex is the last area of the brain to develop in late adolescence to early adulthood, and it is by far the most sophisticated part of the brain. It is the seat of all higher-order mental activity. While it is the most challenging area of the brain to explain, at the same time it is the most exciting. The cortex plays a key role in the experience of chronic pain—and in recovery from chronic pain.

A Historical Perspective

To thoroughly examine the brain's role in how we experience ourselves and the world, we must consider how people throughout history have attempted to answer the question: Where in the body does consciousness reside? Of course, many people have never paused to think about what consciousness even means. For those who have, it might seem obvious that the brain is the source of the "mind" or "consciousness." But that is only because most of us have been taught this from a young age, and because most everything we hear and learn about thinking, feeling, planning, and other conscious activities refers to the brain as their source. But if we go back thousands, or even hundreds, of years when people had little understanding of the body and its internal workings, there would be no basis for people to assume that consciousness resides in the brain. We will find that even the idea of consciousness was a radical conception.

It has been known for thousands of years that we have a consciousness—a mental life—but it was unclear *where* in our body that consciousness was located or where it came from. Even in ancient times, scholars were trying to determine the area of the body in which consciousness or mental life resided. Until recently this was vigorously debated and mostly misunderstood. It was not until the seventeenth and eighteenth centuries that scientists and philosophers began to conclude that specific mental functions had their sources in different areas of the brain. Before this time, other areas of the body, such as the heart and liver, were considered to be responsible for mental activity.

The search for a material basis for consciousness (that is, a location in the body where consciousness could be found) can be traced back at least as far as Hippocrates of Cos, who in the fifth century BC explored the idea that the key to being human is to have a consciousness and the ability to think. Although Hippocrates was unsure where in the body consciousness resided, he claimed that the brain was the organ of the "intellect," or what he called the "guiding spirit." He thought that the heart was the organ of the senses. Thus, Hippocrates gave us the first clue that the brain could be the organ of consciousness and mental life, but he made no attempt to explain how it might work.

About five hundred years later the Greek physician Galen made the first attempt to localize consciousness in the brain. He believed that consciousness resided in the *ventricles*. (Ventricles are fluid-filled chambers inside of the brain just under the *cortex,* the folded outer layer of the brain that, as we mentioned, is the center of our most complex thinking.) Galen believed that there was something special about the fluid that gave us the ability to experience consciousness or mental function. He speculated that special humors were received through the eyes and from the liver and that these humors came together in the fluid of the ventricles to form "psychic humors" or consciousness. (Generally, *humors* were thought to be in bodily fluids; in ancient times, humors such as blood, phlegm, and bile were ascribed various emotional qualities.) Galen's theory may seem primitive now, but at the time it was a radical advancement. He was the first to give the brain an actual function that was responsible for consciousness.

After the concepts of Hippocrates and Galen were proposed, hundreds of years went by with little progress in the search for the material basis of consciousness and the localization of specific functions. Then, in the seventeenth century, scholars began trying to locate the area of the brain where consciousness resided. At this time, they asked if there was a specific area of the brain in which consciousness coincided with the material matter of the brain. The French philosopher René Descartes proposed that a certain gland in the brain, called the pineal gland, was what housed consciousness. Others proposed that consciousness resided in different areas of the brain. This search to find the brain organ or area responsible for our mental life was the first step in what would become the localization of function for specific brain areas.

It was not until the nineteenth century that it became more clear that a relationship existed between consciousness, thought, and brain activity. The German anatomist Franz Joseph Gall in the early 1800s proposed that the gray matter of the cortex housed our mental faculties. He was the first to suggest that mental activity takes place through the actions of brain cells found in the cortex. Gall proposed that specific areas of the cortex were responsible for particular functions such as love of life, the destructive instincts, attentiveness, causality, and imitativeness. Although in modern times we may view Gall's explanation of the brain as naive, it was the first attempt to localize function in the cortex and, in retrospect, was a quite novel and courageous suggestion.

In the mid-1800s, the neurologists Marc Dax and Paul Broca described how damage to a specific area of the cortex could be linked to a loss of specific function. Both described an area of the cortex that they believed was responsible for articulated speech. Broca examined the brain of a man who had a stroke and lost the ability to speak yet was able to comprehend speech perfectly. Broca's discovery stimulated further clinical research that would demonstrate that specific areas of the cortex were associated with other specific functions such as movement, the ability to see, and the ability to feel.

It has always been amazing to me that it took thousands of years for scholars to realize the brain was associated with mental abilities. However, when one considers the state of science and medicine before the scientific revolution that began in the eighteenth century and the mystical-spiritual component that was associated with mental life prior to that, it is not surprising that this development took so long. After all, we did not have the ability to get a clear image of the brain as it functioned in living people until the early 1970s, when the CAT scan was invented. With the radical advances that this technology made possible, it became common knowledge that specific human functions are localized in the cortex. Yet it is still not known specifically how these areas function and interact with one another to create thoughts, feelings, and behaviors. It remains a mystery how consciousness is derived from the workings of a group of nerve cells. However, we have evidence that there is a strong correlation between those nerve cells and the ability to think and have consciousness.

The Structure of the Brain

The brain is made of many specialized cells called *neurons* and *glial cells*. Neurons come together in groups to perform many functions. Networks of neurons form various structures in the brain, including the four lobes and the outer wrapping of the brain, the cortex, which, as noted earlier, is the center of complex thinking. Neurons are supported by specialized cells called glial cells. These provide nutrients, help with metabolism, contain neurotransmitters, and can transmit messages. Though I am not going to go into detail about these structures, some understanding is essential to appreciating how chronic pain can be considered a disease of the brain.

Neurons, synapses, and glial cells

The basic unit of the brain is a specialized cell called a neuron. Neurons are individual nerve cells that have a cell body, a long cylindrical process (an extension of the cell) called an *axon*, and shorter cylindrical processes called *dendrites*. Neurons are able to create an electrical charge and carry an electrical signal. The neuron was not described until the early 1900s, when improved microscopes enabled scientists to look at the brain. Since then, we have made dramatic advances in understanding how neurons function, communicate with one another, and come together to complete tasks.

Neurons interact with each other through a communication process that occurs at a location called the *synapse*. Synapses are tiny gaps between two neurons. Neurons send chemical messages across these gaps. Essentially, the nerve cells exchange chemical substances called *neurotransmitters,* which are released from one end of a neuron and are received, across the synapse, by another neuron. *(See diagram on next page.)*

Neurons come in many different sizes and are able to transmit messages across very large areas. For example, there is an area of the cortex that is responsible for movement. So, to move our big toe, a message must travel from this area of the cortex all the way down to our toe, stimulating the muscles of the toe. Other neurons are much smaller and serve functions such as fine-tuning electric messages within specific areas of the cortex.

Glial cells come in a few different types and help neurons maintain structure and energy. Glial cells also serve other metabolic functions, such as creating and maintaining neurotransmitters. It was recently discovered that these cells are also able to transmit neurotransmitters and may be able to create electrical messages.

Neurons exchange information with other neurons through interactions in the synapse. Scientists now believe that the interaction between neurons and synapses gives us the ability to accomplish psychological functions such as thinking, remembering, planning, and feeling emotions. One of the amazing aspects of the brain and mind is that, we assume,

THE CHEMISTRY OF CELL COMMUNICATION

Neurons carry and process information via electrical signals, which are the basis of communication in the brain. Neurons can be the thought of as wires, since, like wires, they are able to conduct an electrical signal. They are special because they can create an electric charge and transmit it across their cell membrane. They do so by keeping different numbers of charged particles called *ions* across their membrane. Elements such as sodium, potassium, chloride, and calcium are able to hold a charge that is either positive or negative. The neuron creates a charge by holding more negative ions inside of itself compared to the number on the outside. Neurons are able to maintain this charge across the membrane by having channels that act as pumps. These pumps, which require energy in the form of the sugar glucose, carry ions into and out of the neuron. Neurons are also able to conduct messages along the *axons,* which are long, wire-like structures. Other appendages that project from the neuron are called *dendrites*. Dendrites from different neurons interact with each other and are thought to be responsible for much of the processing that occurs between neurons. Both axons and dendrites form synapses with other neurons, and these synapses carry messages between cells. Groups of neurons are able to work together as units.

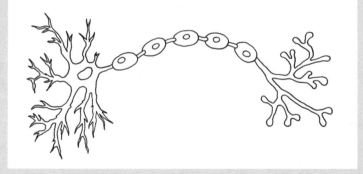

Figure 3. This is a neuron. On the left is the cell body with a circle in the center that represents the nucleus. The appendages coming off of the cell body are dendrites. The longest appendage extending from the cell body is the axon that carries an electrical signal to the right side of the figure where more dendrites are ready to interact with other neurons.

the electrical and chemical processes created in the neurons of the brain are somehow responsible for consciousness and all mental processes. We are far from understanding *how* this comes about, but we do know that when neurons and glial cells are destroyed or do not function properly, consciousness, mental processes, and behavior are dramatically altered. In the case of chronic pain, changes occur in the structure and function of specific groups of neurons. The important thing to remember is that these structural and functional alterations can change back and become normal again thanks to neuroplasticity, the brain's capacity to change itself, which we will explore in more detail in the next chapter, and which is the aim of the exercises in the second part of this book.

Neural networks, lobes, and the cortex

When you and I talk about networks, we think of groups of people concerned about the same activity or cause, or perhaps groups of computers linked together for a common purpose or business. In the brain, groups of neurons work together in a similar way. These *neural networks* are formed by groups of neurons that come together to perform specific tasks. Neural networks are able to interact with other neural networks to access and process information. The interactions that occur between neurons depend on what specific task must be completed.

The activity and interaction of neurons and their ability to come together as units to perform specific tasks and behaviors is one of the wonders of the brain. Neural networks may be restricted to certain parts of the brain or may be spread throughout the nervous system, as with the earlier example of the neural activity involved in moving your big toe. A message is sent from the brain to the spinal cord to a nerve that runs all the way from the spinal cord to the toe. This is done in a very specific, coordinated fashion so that this movement can be carried out with great precision. Importantly, neural networks have the ability to perform multiple tasks. Thus, there is no set limitation on how many tasks a neuron can perform or the number of neural networks that neurons can be involved in.

The cortex (the outer layer of the brain) has distinctive infoldings called *sulci* and outfoldings called *gyri*. These folds allow for more cortical territory—that is, the folded or "compacted" design allows more brain tissue to fit in the same space. As noted earlier, the cortex is the last area of the brain to develop and is the most sophisticated part of the brain. It is where our higher order thought processes occur, such as decision making.

The cortex is composed of two identical halves, called the left hemisphere and right hemisphere. Each hemisphere is a mirror image of the other and is composed of four lobes: the frontal lobe, temporal lobe, parietal lobe, and occipital lobe. Each lobe is associated with specific functions. For example, the main function of the occipital lobe is to process visual information. Each lobe is also able to act as a neural network. However, many neural networks are created *across* multiple lobes and across both hemispheres. This is probably one of the most amazing aspects of the brain—that the collection of nerve cells can join together

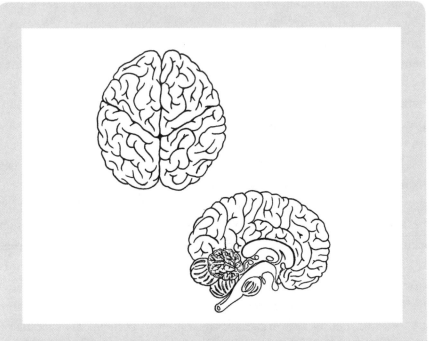

Figure 4. The top figure is a depiction of the two hemispheres of the brain. This is an overhead view in which the left and right cerebral hemispheres of the brain can be seen and are divided by the longitudinal fissure. The left and right frontal lobes are at the top. The bottom figure shows the medial (middle) surface of the left cerebral hemisphere.

to accomplish different tasks, and they can shift duties depending on the task. They can also function as members of different networks—just as you may simultaneously be part of a parents' network, a career network, a civil rights network, an alumni network, and a hobbyist network, serving different functions in each.

The cortex as an information-processing system

The most sophisticated tasks of the human brain are carried out in the cortex. The electrical signals that neurons create and the interactions across synapses are the basis of the brain's ability to process information. Take, for example, the ability to read this page. Information about the words on this page enters your brain through your eyes and is deciphered in the occipital lobe of your brain. Each word has a meaning that is remembered in the brain, probably in the temporal lobe. The brain is able to access these memories of meanings and create strings of meaningful words called sentences that are comprehended and understood. As all of this is going on, you are able to remember what was said in previous sentences, paragraphs, and chapters. This process allows you to put all the information into context so that a story unfolds and the words take on a meaning. You are also able to relate these words to your previous experience and thereby determine how the message is relevant to your life. While this is an abbreviated picture of the human cortex, it gives you a sense of the sophisticated tasks it can accomplish and its important role in processing information.

The cortex is constantly taking in new information, gaining access to remembered information, and often creating new meanings and knowledge that allow us to negotiate our way through life. It is believed that this is being accomplished by the electrical and chemical signals occurring in your brain. Without this ability to take in, remember, access, and create new knowledge, our ability to accomplish goal-directed tasks would be extremely difficult.

It is interesting to imagine that somehow the brain is like a computer that can process information. This analogy is apt in many ways, but there are also problems with it. All computers have been programmed by people for a discrete set of functions, and this creates limitations on what they are able to accomplish. The programmers program computers with certain tasks in mind, such as performing calculations or decoding and processing large bodies of data. In contrast, the human cortex has the ability to create new programs as it goes along. This ability and the action itself depends on what environmental stimulation the human cortex experiences. Thus there is an aspect of creativity to the human cortex that is lacking in the computer.

When a computer breaks, you are stuck—the computer is not going to fix itself. That is another wonderful difference between a computer and the cortex: the human cortex has the ability to change and improve and, in a sense, heal itself. We assume that in order to do this the cortex must be able to auto-regulate (or rewrite) its programming. *The brain's amazing capacity to reprogram itself is especially relevant because it is this capacity that will help you overcome chronic pain.*

The Brain Cortex in Pain

In earlier chapters, we described some of the behavioral and cognitive changes that occur when people experience chronic pain. Over the last two decades it has become increasingly clear that as pain becomes chronic, the neurons and neural networks change. We assume that, as the structure and function of the neurons and neural networks change, there is also a change in the perceptions, thoughts, attention, and behavior of the individual. In the case of chronic pain, the areas of the brain affected are the frontal lobe, the temporal lobe, and the parietal lobe.

Chronic pain appears to affect the individual neurons and the synapses by which these neurons communicate. Areas of the brain that are involved in attention and goal-directed behavior are altered, and the neurons involved in these processes become less able to function properly. Areas that keep negative emotions in check are also altered. With the condition of chronic pain, other areas of the brain that focus our attention on pain, generate negative emotions, cause us to ruminate on negative thoughts, keep us anxious, and disrupt our sleep become more active. The good news about these changes is that they have occurred as a result of environmental stimulation and, as will be seen in the next chapter, we can alter that stimulation so these brain areas can revert to their previous form and function normally again.

The frontal lobe is another very sophisticated area of the brain. It is the area where final decisions are made after all of the information from other areas of the brain has been processed and considered. If one were to make an analogy to a ship, the frontal lobe of the brain would be where the captain would sit, giving the navigator directions about where the ship should go. The frontal lobe of the brain has the ability to focus attention on those aspects of the internal and external environment that allow one to accomplish goal-directed tasks. As we have learned, with chronic pain this ability becomes considerably diminished as attention is shifted away from goal-directed behavior and placed on the sensation of pain. This occurs because there are structural and functional alterations in the frontal lobe.

One important part of the frontal lobe is the *orbital frontal cortex*. This area of the brain has two important tasks. One is to give the captain of the ship the most important option (the priority) in order to accomplish the task the individual seeks to accomplish. The other important job is to block out all negative emotions. But the ability to accomplish this task declines with chronic pain. There is also a dramatic and overwhelming flood of negative emotions that occur with chronic pain. It is as though the captain of the ship, distracted by haunting memories of pain, cannot stay focused on critical activities, such as avoiding another ship.

Another area of the cortex that is important with chronic pain is located between the frontal lobe and temporal lobe. Called the *insular cortex,* this area of the cortex essentially maps out the environment inside the body. Through the work of the insular cortex, we gain information about the location of the body, how an area of the body feels, and, most important, any emotional aspects associated with that area of the body. In patients with chronic pain this area of the brain is extremely overactive. The insular cortex in these patients is more focused on unpleasant feelings in some area of the body and the negative emotions associated with that area. As a result, people with chronic pain constantly pay attention to the negative feelings occurring inside their body.

The areas of the cortex that regulate chronic stress, fear, and anxiety also lose proper function in people with chronic pain. As a result, the stress response becomes chronic and ongoing. The person continually experiences both fear over anticipated pain and unremitting ruminations on pain.

Conclusion

The study of the brain has a long and difficult history. Even the now seemingly obvious understanding that the brain is associated with consciousness was a very long time in coming. As philosophers and scientists worked to develop and test ideas, they gradually learned some of the functions and processes of the brain.

We know now that neurons are the basic building blocks of the brain. They communicate across synapses via electrical signals, using chemicals called neurotransmitters, and are supported by a type of cell called glial cells. Neural networks, groups of nerve cells that come together, create processes that enable us to accomplish tasks. The same neuron can be part of a variety of different networks. These networks are assembled in various parts of the brain, including the left and right hemispheres, each of which has a frontal lobe, temporal lobe, occipital lobe, and parietal lobe.

The most sophisticated part of the human brain is the cortex—the outer part of the brain made up of infoldings and outfoldings. This part of the brain is where we do most of our thinking, emotional processing, and other important tasks of mental life, reflection, and self-regulation. When we experience chronic pain, certain areas of the cortex are changed, causing us to shift attention and focus from goals and tasks to the negative feelings, fear, and anxiety related to pain. Fortunately, the brain can rewrite the "programs" that have been altered by chronic pain. In the next chapter, I will detail how changes occur in the nerve cells of neural networks.

• • •

6

Neuroplasticity

When I was a kid, I decided I wanted train to be an athlete. I was going to dedicate time each day to accomplish this endeavor. I went to a Saturday morning sports camp where a college football coach talked about beginning a daily routine to improve performance. I soon recognized that such a routine could help me build my endurance and strength. I would improve my cardiovascular system, lung function, and speed. I knew I could build muscle, improve attention, and increase knowledge of any sport I chose by exercising and practicing specific skills. Essentially then, by doing proper exercise, I could start to realize whatever potential I had.

Although I understood that I could do that with my body, at the time *I had no idea that it was possible to do the same process with my brain.* Today I know that the skill and exercise routine was also improving my brain. Moreover, improving my brain was probably the most important part of that routine. As a child, I had no knowledge of a process that today we call *neuroplasticity,* nor did I know that, in a sense, one could build "brain muscle" (neuron structure and processing strength) just as one builds body muscle. I still find it remarkable that my youthful interest in athletic strength and skill training would one day translate to my life's work designing and overseeing a program for people with chronic pain and addiction based on theories about neuroplasticity!

Neuroplasticity—the brain's capacity to change itself—is a hot topic these days. A quick Internet search delivers a multitude of websites offering methods to improve brain function through neuroplasticity. All claim that engaging in their methods will improve brain health by adding more "muscle" to the brain (or something like that). Advertised methods range from physical exercise, to puzzles and games, to amino acids for daily consumption, to "nine easy steps to neuroplasticity." I even came across a website that offered neuroplasticity for children. I found this one especially interesting because the child's brain is *already* constantly going through neuroplastic changes, since it is in the process of development. I guess the people behind that site think it is possible to speed up or improve this process.

You would be right to be skeptical of all these Web offerings. However, neuroplasticity is a serious topic, and within the last decade we have made tremendous progress in understanding how the brain constantly changes when it is stimulated. Still, the study of neuroplasticity is in its infancy— one reason to approach Internet offers with skepticism. Although we have learned much, there is much yet to discover. In this chapter, you will learn about the basic principles of neuroplasticity and how it is relevant to the treatment of chronic pain.

Our Changing Brain

I want to review some of the information from the last chapter, because these are complex concepts that are not always easy to take in from one reading. The way we have discovered this information is fascinating, and I will tell some of that story as well in this chapter, but let's begin by going over some basics. Remember, you do not have to memorize all the technical terms presented here; the important thing is to make the connection between how the brain functions, including its capacity to change, and how you experience and deal with chronic pain.

Here are five important things to remember about the brain that will lay the foundation for our discussion of neuroplasticity:

1. The human brain is composed of about 100 billion neurons. Neurons, as discussed in the previous chapter, are nerve cells that are the basic building blocks of the brain. Neurons have long (from a cellular perspective) branches called axons and dendrites, and they communicate via chemicals called neurotransmitters that are passed across synapses, or spaces between neurons. In essence, they are passing electrical signals through the brain and body. Amazingly, neurons can assemble into neural networks that can process information, and they can serve in more than one network. In a sense, our brain functions as a very complex computer with unheard-of processing ability.

2. You may recall from chapter 1 that though our brain is the information "processing unit," we have another phenomenon that we call our mind that gives us consciousness. The mind seems to be associated with the brain, and it is like a movie telling the story of our lives. It is also continually interpreting the information our brain collects. It is thought that the ability to have a mind and consciousness somehow emerges from the workings and interactions of those 100 billion neurons that make up our brain, but we have much to learn about this. We do know that the ability of those neurons to process information efficiently results in more useful and adaptive mental states.

3. Each neuron has the ability to either grow or contract depending on the environmental stimulation it has been exposed to. If a certain area of the brain is stimulated and needs to process information better, it can grow. Through stimulation, neurons can either improve or decrease their function by changing their structure. For example, a neuron can add more dendrites when it becomes stimulated. These dendrites can improve both the neuron's processing ability and the amount of communication it has with other neurons.

4. Growing means adding more processing units, either dendrites or synapses, or changing how the synapses function.

5. When I use the word *environment* I mean either our external environment (what we perceive from the outside world) or our internal environment (what we perceive from inside of ourselves). It is important to make this distinction because when we talk about stress, much of the bad stress that is created when we are in pain comes from inside of ourselves, especially our thoughts.

From these five statements it should be clear that our brain (and, for that matter, every nerve cell in our brain) is in a constant state of change. This change occurs in the brain's structure (physical appearance) and the brain's function (the things it can do) as it responds to its internal and external environment. The structure and function of our brain have a direct effect on our mind, mental states, and consciousness—our personal "narrative."

If you understand this, it is time to move on to define neuroplasticity. If any of this is not quite clear, give yourself all the time you need to take the information in.

> **Neuroplasticity** is the brain's ability to change structure and function as a way of adapting to an ever-changing internal and external environment.

Neuroplasticity can be extraordinarily helpful, as it allows us to adapt to new challenges. For example, consider the skills you had to develop just to get around in the adult world. You probably had to learn how to read bus schedules or determine the best driving routes to get where you needed to go. Now these tasks are automatic, because your brain has practiced the skills until they became routine.

On the other hand, neuroplasticity can be very unhelpful if the changes occur in areas of the brain that make you more anxious or unable to turn off the stress response, as may occur with an anxiety disorder.

Therefore, it is important to understand that the key issue is where and how neuroplasticity occurs. When one develops chronic pain, important areas of the brain have changed, and these changes take attention away from ordinary life and place it on pain and its effects, including the fear of feeling it.

The Discovery and Understanding of Neuroplasticity

You have no doubt heard the very old saying "You can't teach an old dog new tricks." Scientists have a habit of asking questions about these sorts of long-held beliefs. Today, we have proven that this ancient "wisdom" should be packed away next to the notion of a flat earth (which is not to say that there aren't times when it is *easier* to learn new tricks).

In the late 1960s and 1970s the Nobel laureates David Hubel and Torsten Wiesel began studying the visual system. Their research explained a lot about how the visual system is able to perceive light from the environment and how the visual system develops by interacting with the visual environment. Perhaps their most important finding was that there is a particular period of time in our development during which the visual system develops the ability to perceive depth. It seemed that if information from the environment does not reach the visual system by a specific point in our early development, the visual system will not develop normally. This period of early development, during which the visual system is especially susceptible to environmental deprivation, is called a *critical period.* Hubel and Wiesel's research was important because it demonstrated that the brain had a particular period during which neuroplastic changes could occur. It appeared that after this period, the brain became fixed and could not continue to change—at least in terms of the visual system.

Similar critical periods were described for the somatosensory system (feeling) and the olfactory system (smell). I was fortunate to have been part of the team that discovered a similar period for the sense of taste when I worked with Dave Hill at the University of Virginia as a PhD candidate. We were able to identify a period of early prenatal development when the taste system could be altered. We characterized this as a *sensitive period* and went on with a colleague, Doug Mook, to describe how the taste system could very rapidly return to normal when the environment shifted from an altered state back to normal.

At the time I did not realize this was a neuroplastic ability—that is, that the brain's sense of taste could be altered and then, after an environmental change, become normal again. I often go back to this research experience when I am thinking about how the environment must change to improve brain function and help people with chronic pain.

So, early studies seemed to show that the brain "fixed," or set, certain abilities at specific times—in a sense, supporting the idea that you can't teach an old dog new tricks. Yet the research I was fortunate to participate in showed that at least one capacity—taste—was able to change. Other studies have shown that great changes are possible in other areas when the brain is exposed to new experiences.

To date, the best known example of neuroplastic changes that the brain undergoes with experience was described in a study of London taxi drivers. London taxi drivers go through extensive pre-employment training. They learn the streets of London and the shortest routes from one destination to another. Researchers found that by the time the taxi drivers completed this training, their brains were actually larger than before. Indeed, the area of the taxi driver's brain responsible for spatial memory became significantly larger in volume. That is, cortical gray matter increased in the spatial memory area of the brain after these taxi drivers had undergone route training. The implication was, of course, that the training was responsible for the increase in gray matter and that the increase in gray matter meant more memory and processing ability for driving the routes of London. There was no other plausible explanation: the changes occurred specifically in the area of the brain involved with spatial memory, and the increase in size was associated with the pre-employment training. This was an exciting finding because it revealed that even in the adult brain, environmental experience can dramatically alter and enhance the brain and its function. In other words, an old dog can indeed learn new tricks.

Since the study on the London taxi drivers, many other studies have shown both positive and negative results from neuroplastic changes in the brain. Many studies have investigated the neuroplastic changes that occur with common diseases such as depression, anxiety, schizophrenia, and chronic pain. These studies have found changes in both the structure and function of the brain with these diseases when compared to normal brains. In the case of chronic pain, significant neuroplastic changes occur in important areas of the brain that regulate such functions as the stress response, attention, decision making, emotions, and attention to internal states. Most important, one study has shown that when chronic pain is properly treated, the neuroplastic changes experienced with chronic pain can be reversed. This is exciting because it demonstrates that with proper treatment, these changes are alterable.

Neuroplasticity and Chronic Pain

Perhaps the easiest way to understand neuroplasticity is to think of a computer. You have a computer that can perform many tasks but there are certain tasks you would like it to perform that it cannot. There are a number of options available to you. One option would be to add processing ability to the computer so that it can easily accomplish what you want. This would involve adding new circuits to your computer in the form of microchips. After this is done (and if it is done properly), the computer can perform the tasks you wanted. In a similar fashion, if proper neuroplasticity occurs, you can enhance your brain function and accomplish processing information that was previously outside your capacity.

With a computer, we change the processing ability by adding circuits or changing programming. With the brain, we change processing ability through environmental stimulation. This may include practicing new routines (think of the London taxi drivers), learning to quiet your mind, finding ways to get the stress response under control, and practicing taking control of your attention. Such practices may rewire the areas of the brain in charge of these skills and enable them to perform better. Let's explore how this might apply to the brain of someone who has chronic pain.

If you have chronic pain, it is not hard to understand that many of your thoughts are couched with negative content, and that causes fear and anxiety. Everything seems shaded by persistent discomfort. This makes living difficult, which in the language of brain development means that the response is *maladaptive.* That is, rather than helping you live a productive, positive life, your brain's responses interfere with your ability to do that. One explanation for this phenomenon is that the areas of the brain that should control these maladaptive responses have been altered by pain. Let's take a look at how that may work.

I have previously explained how memories of pain (or previous experiences of pain) can construct the foundation for a future of chronic physical pain. Part of the problem is that the areas of the brain that control the stress response have been markedly altered. The past negative events (or a collection of negative events over time) activated the stress response, which is commonly called the *fight-or-flight response.* The response activates a number of chemicals and conditions in the body that puts us in a tense, highly alert state. The conditions are helpful for a short time—like when we need to fight or flee from someone who is threatening us or when we need to deal with another real, immediate crisis. But when these conditions persist for a long time, they are damaging to the body. Because of this, when the stress response is initiated, parallel processes begin that will rapidly turn it off to protect that body.

When people have repeated adverse experiences, especially as children, the stress response becomes more active. In time, it also becomes easier to turn on and harder and harder to turn off. In some cases, it may not be possible to turn it off at all. This means that when a person is in chronic pain, there is constant stress. So, if you have had a lot of adversity in your life or if you have been under a tremendous amount of stress, you have established the foundation for chronic pain. Then when chronic pain occurs, it just adds to and intensifies your stress.

This state has occurred because the neuroplastic changes in the areas of the brain that control the stress response—the prefrontal cortex and hippocampus—diminish the ability of these areas to actually control the response and areas of the brain that initiate the stress response—such as the amygdala—dominate. As a result, important areas of the prefrontal cortex become affected. To understand these effects, we need to return to more brain anatomy.

My apologies to those of you who do not enjoy science. However, I am not going into this detail just because it is fascinating to me. I have learned from my patients that as they begin to understand how their brain works, they begin the process of healing. As you will see repeatedly in this book, recovery from chronic pain involves retraining the brain, which requires some knowledge of how it works!

Toward the end of the previous chapter, we talked about an area of the brain called the insular cortex. To recap, this area of the brain is involved in surveying how the body feels internally. It gives you a map of the internal state of your body, not just in terms of sensations and their location, but also in terms of how those sensations are being interpreted in the context of the current narrative (your personal "movie" about your life). For example, the insular cortex helps you sort through sensations and answer the question, Is that a sensation I associate with pain and how does that sensation affect my tendency toward negative thoughts, hypervigilance, or rumination? In patients with chronic pain, the insular cortex becomes overactive. It has undergone neuroplastic changes that have caused it to process too many internal sensations that are associated with negative emotions. The brain's ability to focus on other important aspects of life has been hijacked by paying too much attention to potentially painful sensations. Attention is focused on how the body does not feel well and what the mind thinks about that (that is, how the message "my body does not feel well" fits into your personal narrative). The brain also becomes hypervigilant to any internal sensations and begins to label all of them as negative and painful. What might have once felt like a tired or slightly stretched muscle now feels deeply painful. What may have once felt like a mildly upset stomach is now interpreted as pain. These changes occur as the insular cortex and the mind's interpretation of its messages become stuck in a rut that sends every signal down the pain path. Thus any treatment program for chronic pain must address these neuroplastic changes, and the treatment must include a component that helps them return to normal, adaptive function.

Another area of the brain is called the *dorsolateral prefrontal cortex*. In the previous chapter, we used the analogy of the brain as a ship in need of a captain; the dorsolateral prefrontal cortex is the area where the captain and navigator would work. This is the area of the brain where the final decisions are made after all available information has been collected and analyzed. One of the important jobs of the dorsolateral prefrontal cortex is to turn off the pain response. In the normal brain this is accomplished in a short amount of time through a network of neurons that has the ability to alter the pain response and shut it off. Studies have shown that both the structure and function of the dorsolateral prefrontal cortex are altered by pain. With chronic pain, this area of the brain undergoes neuroplastic changes and can no longer keep focused on important aspects of the internal and external environment that allow one to accomplish goal-directed tasks. Instead, attention has been captured by pain and decisions are being made through the lens that has been formed by the constant experience of pain. Pain catastrophizing (the tendency to assume or predict the worst outcome), attention to pain, and the perceived inability to achieve goals become exaggerated, while the ability to turn the pain signal off becomes compromised.

Interestingly, this "pain response control" ability in the dorsolateral prefrontal cortex that is altered in chronic pain *is also altered with chronic opioid use*. And in order for chronic pain to be properly treated, this area of the brain must experience *positive* neuroplastic changes so it can regain control.

NEUROPLASTICITY AND OPIOIDS

In chapter 3, we discussed maladaptive changes that occur with chronic exposure to opioids. As you may recall, opioids interact with specific receptors in the brain to help dull pain. After the opioids have interacted with these receptors, a number of changes occur inside the brain cell that help turn down the signal of pain. Chronic opioid use can cause opioid receptors, such as the mu receptor, to undergo a number of neuroplastic changes. For example, we mentioned earlier that chronic opioid use causes the number of opioid receptors to decrease (a process that is referred to as *down regulation*). Literally, the number of opioid receptors in the cell membrane is reduced. This reduction, in turn, diminishes the cell's ability to respond to the opioids. When this happens, the person may perceive either a reduced ability of the drug to produce its former effect (tolerance) or an increase in pain (hyperalgesia).

Another neuroplastic change that occurs with chronic opioid use is *desensitization.* This occurs when opioid receptors become less able to activate the second messenger (molecules that relay signals from receptors on the cell surface to target molecules inside the cell). Again, the result is a much less effective opioid.

Still another neuroplastic change is *counteradaptation.* Here the amount of perceived pain in the brain is increased through chronic opiate use. This may happen as a result of increased excitation of those areas of the brain that produce the sensation of pain and all of its associated misery.

As can be seen from these examples, chronic opioid use leads to striking changes in the brain. None of them are positive changes, and all involve altering the structure and function of important areas involved in the processing of opioids. These are among many reasons why I do not think opioids are a good choice for the treatment of chronic pain.

The *medial prefrontal cortex,* which processes risk and fear, is another important area of the brain that undergoes structural and functional changes with chronic pain. These alterations cause chronic pain patients to keep their attention on pain and all the negative emotions associated with it. In the normal brain, the medial prefrontal cortex will take control over these negative emotions and thereby allow the dorsolateral prefrontal cortex to make optimal decisions. But with chronic pain, this ability is compromised and negative emotions prevail.

The medial prefrontal cortex also plays an important role in presenting a number of options to the dorsolateral prefrontal cortex in order to accomplish a given goal-directed task. In chronic pain patients, this ability is also altered through neuroplasticity and so the choices that are made are often suboptimal, such as choosing to not exercise and otherwise carry on a healthy lifestyle. So not only is the captain of the brain—the dorsolateral prefrontal cortex—compromised, but so is its primary tactical officer. The captain is distracted by pain and will not make decisions, while the tactical officer cannot come up with decent options to get the ship on the right course.

These are a few examples of how neuroplastic alterations in the structure and function of the brain cause chaos for people with chronic pain. In the second part of this book, you will learn exercises to help you overcome and change these maladaptive neuroplastic changes.

Conclusion

I hope this discussion has helped you understand and appreciate neuroplasticity—the basic idea that the brain changes with environmental stimulation. People with chronic pain may have experienced significant neuroplastic changes in the brain that eventually led to their chronic pain and all the associated misery. The good news is that through proper treatment and stimulation, this can be altered.

Some of the information in this chapter is obviously theoretical—that is, we have strong evidence that it is the case but have not yet proven it conclusively. This uncertainty is because we do not currently have the ability to map how one goes from a state of functioning brain neurons to a state of consciousness. In other words, we still do not understand how all those things that go on in the brain assemble into the thing we call our mind. We take the liberty to assume that because there is a correlation between mental states and alterations in brain structure and function, the alteration in physical tissue and conceptual mental states are somehow causing each other. That is an honest analysis—we just do not know the full answer to this yet. But that does not mean we cannot use what we have learned about the brain's amazing capacity to change itself (for good or for bad results) to help ourselves find relief from chronic pain. The methods you learn moving forward do not prove that I am "right." But, it is encouraging that they work and are beginning to be supported by research.

The next chapter will be about the *mind*. I have been slowly introducing this concept and have indicated that it plays a key role in everything that goes on with the experience of chronic pain. I have studied the mind for many years and will describe some important aspects of it that are relevant to the treatment of chronic pain. Indeed, it is a challenge to try to describe the mind and consciousness as an independent entity because, frankly, *it has no material extension*. That is to say, I cannot point to a specific place in my body and say, "My mind exists here" with any degree of confidence. But, for me, that is what makes it exciting and worthwhile to study.

· · ·

7

The Mind

For thousands of years, philosophers, theologians, and scientists have been studying the mind and have written volumes on the topic. This is not surprising, considering that the mind is the vehicle by which you are able to be conscious. For example, as you read and understand the words in this book, reflect on what they mean, and consider how this meaning may apply to your life, all of this is occurring because you have a mind. Indeed, the mind enables us to be conscious of the world, of ourselves, and of past and future experience. It constitutes the very essence of our existence.

Most of the work that has examined the mind has been aimed at explaining what the mind *is*. Certain aspects of the mind, such as consciousness, perception, judgment, reasoning, attention, and memory, are often studied. Throughout the history of the philosophy of mind, and still today, there have been a number of mysteries that have caused much speculation and many arguments. For example, philosophers have continued to wonder about the correspondence between the outside world (what we perceive that exists outside our body) and our ability to represent that world in our mind. Many have wondered about the relationship between perception and how that perception is interpreted in our mind. Some have argued that there is a direct correspondence between what actually exists in the world and what our mind is able to represent. Still others have argued that there is an indirect correspondence between what exists in the world and what our mind represents. That is to say, there is little connection between what physically exists in the world and the information that comes into our mind after it is processed.

Another common area of disagreement involves the relationship between mind and body. *Monists* argue that the mind and body are the same and that both are made from the same elements and atoms that make up all other things in the world. *Dualists* argue that the mind and body are separate entities and there is something special about the mind that cannot be captured by the same laws that govern elements and atoms.

For the purposes of this book and this chapter, I will assume that there is a correspondence between what exists in the world and what we are able to represent about the world in our mind. This is referred to as *correspondence theory*. It states that while it does not always happen, we are capable of representing in our mind what actually exists in the world. I will also assume that there is a direct relationship between things we are able to represent in our mind and the meaning we give to them. This means that the things we are able to represent in our mind are directly related to things in the world and, to the extent that this relationship represents reality, it is true.

At first, it may seem strange that I am beginning a chapter about the mind in a book on chronic pain by discussing historical debates that have occurred for thousands of years. As a person wanting some practical answers about your chronic pain, you may be wondering if any of this really matters. But it does, because we often take these arguments for granted and do not even take the time to ask these kinds of questions about our own lives. I have found that it is important to think about these ideas in terms of *how we experience pain as a way of being in the world* if we are to understand how we can begin a path toward conquering chronic pain.

Consider the nature of what you perceive and how pain may have changed your perception of the world and of yourself. For example, it will be important that you begin to think about what you perceive, how you process your perceptions, and how pain of any sort may have changed or skewed the representation of reality that you have in your mind. Similarly, when you begin to work on the exercises in part 2, your ability to analyze what you perceive and what your mind is doing will be very important. You must be willing and able to begin a journey of self-inquiry that includes considering the nature of mind and consciousness. *That* is why this chapter should matter to you!

In this chapter, I will highlight parts of the vast and important research on the mind and relate some of the important ideas from the philosophy of mind. I will also describe aspects of what we understand about how the mind works so that in future chapters you will see how your mind has been altered by pain. As you read on, this information will help you understand how these aspects of the philosophy of mind will enable you to overcome pain. First, mind is important because it is where we experience both the world around us and the world inside of us. It is also the place where we experience pain as first merely a sensation and then as an interpretation with certain meanings that can have a dramatic impact on our lives. As someone with chronic pain, you may interpret that sensation in a way that gets you into trouble, as it is generally quite negative and couched in suffering and fear.

What Is Mind?

From what we concluded after looking at the history of mind, I think we can agree that it is our mind that gives us the ability to represent the world, not only from moment to moment, but also for long periods of time, even for many years. Part of this comes from our ability to recall memories preserved from our past experience, often with great detail. Besides being able to experience the present and remember our past, we have the ability to project our imagination into the future and determine with some detail what we expect the future to be or what we want the future to be (or do not want it to be). Our mind has the ability to do all of these things. So with those basic assumptions, let's put a definition to *mind*.

> *Mind* constitutes a complex set of abilities (functions) that allow us to perceive and allow us the ability to create concepts (to have thoughts).

Put another way, our mind allows us to be conscious and to be aware of the external and internal environment. The mind's job is to explain the world and put it into an understandable sequence. To do this, our mind must possess the ability to create a unified stream of consciousness that brings together our thoughts from moment to moment and puts them into a *narrative* (an ongoing story) that is understandable and explains the world. This narrative or "world explanation" is one of the primary abilities of our mind. Such congruity helps us interpret the things we see in the world as well as the things we think about, whether those things are imagined or real. In other words, mind enables us to arrange our thoughts into a sequence and create a story (the narrative) of what we are perceiving or thinking about.

In order for this narrative to be accurate, there must be some correspondence between the things that exist in the world and the things we perceive. As we create our narrative, we give meanings to this correspondence. For example, if we encounter a tree in our yard, we perceive a solid object that we have all agreed corresponds to what we mean by the word *tree*. This correspondence between what is perceived and the meaning we give it is referred to as *semantics* (meanings). The meanings we assign to things must correspond in some way to the truth about what is happening in the world or what has happened in the past. We arrive at a truth by having our meanings confirmed by other people. So, we perceive things and make sense of them through an ongoing narrative that consists of our interpretation of the words that is understandable and shared by others. We get a sense that the meanings and narrative we have created are effective when we can interpret present events, use these interpretations to plan (successfully) for future events, and accurately recall past ones.

I have been using the word *meaning* as though we all agreed on its "meaning"! It is a key concept, so let's spend a little more time examining meaning.

Meaning

The mind has the ability to assign meaning to internal and external experiences. *Meaning* refers to the way we interpret the things we experience, perceive, or imagine. For example, each word you are reading has a meaning that, for the most part, is reasonably clear because of convention—most people use that word in the same way. These meanings enable us to communicate with each other through spoken word, written word, or sign language. The statements that we use in our language generally are true or false depending on how they correspond to the state of affairs in the world we share with others of similar psychological, historical, and cultural perspectives.

We have the ability to store meanings and learn new meanings at any time. We also have the ability to change and reinterpret meanings—for example, what we thought was true previously may take on a new meaning or truth. We can also learn to appreciate that people of another time or culture might assign different meanings to the same experience, statement, or even the same word.

Most of us agree there is a physical world that exists outside of us and independent of our perceiving it. We have direct access to the world through our perception of it. These statements may seem obvious or trivial, but they have been debated by philosophers and psychologists for thousands of years. Some philosophers have even questioned if the world actually exists outside of our perceiving it. Others have asked if we are really capable of perceiving the world as it exists or if the world is simply an illusion, since all of the information processed through our senses enters our consciousness and is interpreted by the mind.

These discussions are tied to the concept of *perception*—the way we sense our surrounding world and inner world. Let's now turn to the question of perception. What does it actually mean to be able to perceive?

Perception

Few of us would question that we are able to perceive the world through our senses. We are able to use vision, touch, hearing, taste, and smell as well as internal sensations to experience the world. Each time we experience the world through our senses, we experience a sensation before our mind interprets it. For example, you are sensing the words on this page as changes in light. Before your mind can give the words meaning, they are simply sensations. If you have background music on, music comes into your mind as sound waves that are converted to electrical signals and are perceived as sound in the brain. The sound is simply a sensation until you realize (or interpret) that it is indeed your favorite Beethoven symphony or Beatles song. If you divert your eyes away from the page and direct your attention to the wall, you will notice that the wall is a color. The sensation of that color occurs before your mind gives it meaning or interpretation, such as "That wall is orange, my favorite color." The lesson here is critical: *sensations come before interpretations.* Sensations come into our mind and are given meanings. These meanings are assembled to create our narrative.

Sensations are made up of *qualia.* Qualia are the properties of a sensation available only by one's private direct experience. For example, if I look at the sky, I see it as a particular shade of blue. That blue color is a quality of the sensation of the sky and is one of the qualia that is available to my attention. Qualia are the elemental pieces that make up a sensation. Few of us take the time to pay attention to the qualia that are available to us. We tend to focus on the meaning or interpretation that we have given to the sensation. Generally, the meaning or interpretation has an emotional tag. This is especially true of the internal sensation we call pain. For example, you may be experiencing the sensation of pain, but as will become clear, you are experiencing more than simply a sensation. That is because sensations, on their own, have no interpretation. They are simply the product of a collection of qualia that we are able to perceive.

As we move forward in this book, I will ask you to analyze the qualia that are available to you. You will find when the exercises begin that the most important qualia are those that occur when you direct your attention to what is going on inside of you. That is, "What sensations are available inside my body and what are the qualia of those sensations?" You must become willing to practice putting your attention on them and learn to relieve the burden associated with those sensations.

Each perception has a *phenomenal character.* Phenomenal character is a term used by philosophers to describe what it is like for you personally to undergo the experience of having that sensation. Phenomenal character is the narrative story of the particular sensation. This occurs when we attach a meaning to the sensation and incorporate it into an ongoing narrative. Our personal interpretation of phenomenal characters is largely a product of our past experience, which influences how we process present information. As you will see, your personal phenomenal character of pain is what determines how that pain influences your life. This is why it is important to analyze why a particular sensation has a particular meaning.

So far, we have seen that sensations and meanings are important to the creation of our narrative—the story that our mind unfolds to make sense of the world. But to make sense of what things mean, it is essential that we have memory. Memory is the ability to store information. Let's examine memory and its role in the creation of our narrative.

Memory

The mind has the ability to remember and store information. We rely on this inborn ability to bring unity and clarity to the world. Memory allows us to learn things about the world and ourselves and to later recall them. There are many ways of approaching memory, but for the purposes of this chapter I will divide memory into four types: working memory, semantic memory, episodic memory, and autobiographical memory.

Working memory is the memory you use from moment to moment, such as when you are reading this book. It enables you to remember what has occurred in the recent past, how it relates to what is happening in the present, and how that can be put into a stream of consciousness that makes sense. Working memory allows you to store and process information and combine it with new incoming information. Your mind combines these current and stored pieces of information into an ongoing conscious experience of the world.

Semantic memory allows you to give meaning to objects and experiences in the world, and eventually to life itself. For instance, if you are sitting in a chair, you know that *chair* has the meaning of "something that will hold me while I read a book, rest, or meditate." The chair may also take on special functional meanings, such as something you can stand on to change the lightbulb or to help you to escape a fire by using it to break through a window. Semantic memory is characterized by meanings that help us make sense of our lives, and these meanings can be stored and called up when needed.

Episodic memory is the memory of specific episodes in your life, such as what happened on a specific date or with a specific person. We often have very vivid memories of episodes from our lives that include the emotions attached to the temperature, the season, the time of day, and even smells and tastes connected with those memories. For example, the smell of cookies baking may summon fond memories of an episode of making cookies with a parent.

Autobiographical memory is probably the most important memory that we will discuss. It is the collective memory that is the story of your life. It is memory of the person you are in the world and the story you remember, as far back as you can, of who you are. The autobiographical memory creates an *autobiographical narrative* that is part of your working memory, giving you the essence of "self" as you move through life. When you are in chronic pain, the autobiographical narrative often takes on special meaning, because certain events that are part of your autobiographical narrative are contributing to pain. If you suffer from chronic pain, your present autobiographical narrative has the "flavor" of pain.

Attention

Attention is the ability of the mind to choose important aspects of either the internal or external environment and make them the priority. Certain aspects of the environment are said to be *salient,* which means they are the best choice for giving the mind the ability to complete goal-directed behavior. Attention should be under the control of the individual. This means you should have the ability to focus your attention on anything that you want to. It should be by choice, or volition. Attention is an essential aspect of mind because it allows you to *choose which aspects of perception you want to attend to*. For example, a person in a busy train station may choose to tune out the surrounding noise and foot traffic and read a magazine. She has placed her attention on the magazine. For people with chronic pain, this ability has been diminished or lost. Fortunately, the capacity can be reclaimed through practice.

Awareness

Besides meaning, perception, memory, and attention, another essential component of the mind is awareness, and I give it special importance because awareness is the key to unlocking and releasing the burden of chronic pain. We typically think that being "aware" of something means that it has your attention. In this usual sense of the word, we might be aware that we are sitting, looking at a dog, reading, listening to music, or whatever. But for the purpose of this book, *awareness* has a different meaning. It is a unique aspect of mind that may be experienced during a meditative state. As I use the term, awareness has a more transcendent quality. It is the capacity to be purely conscious without any interpretation of the outside world or internal sensations. You can think of awareness as the process of observing the mind itself without judgment, interpretation, emotional response, or other baggage.

Awareness is a skill, and it is one every person can develop. Developing the skill of awareness will be a major goal of the exercises in part 2 of the book. Pure awareness will help you "clear" the burden that is keeping you in pain—that is, you will not remove the memory or experience, but you will no longer let it drive your attention.

Self-referential awareness

Self-referential awareness is a unique aspect of awareness. The term describes our mind's ability to perceive while simultaneously knowing that there is a "self" (a person) doing the perceiving. I know it sounds complex, but please hang in there with me. Self-referential awareness has been discussed for many years by psychologists, philosophers, and neuroscientists. Considered an essential aspect of what the mind can do, it involves how one is aware of oneself and the perspective one takes to relate to that awareness. *Self-referential awareness is an essential part of our mind, and so understanding it is a part of recovery from chronic pain.*

Our mind has the ability to perform self-related representations. By this I mean that we are able to refer to ourselves, know that we are the perceiver, and have some idea of who we are. One way of understanding this is to understand what is meant by *I*-related and *Me*-related self-reference. I have created these constructs as a way to represent the two aspects of self that we all experience as the *objective-observer self* that we mean when we say "I," and the *subjective self* that we mean when we say "Me." (These may be difficult concepts at first, but as you read they will become much more clear.) First, let's understand the *I* perspective.

I is the *perceiver*. The *I* is the one who perceives both the inner and outer world and is able to represent these perceptions in the mind. However, the *I* in this model is the *objective self* who does not interpret perceptions but is simply aware of the interpretations that are collectively represented in the mind as the *subjective self,* or *Me. I* is the observer:

I perceives the world, as well as the *Me* as a part of the world (what we commonly experience as self-consciousness), as an observer who does not have a subjective interpretation of that perception. The *I* only loses its objectivity when it identifies with the *Me*. When that happens, the *I* disappears into the subjective self that interprets all perceptions based on the limited, emotionally driven perspective of the *autobiographical narrative.* However, when the *I* is not identifying with the *Me* and is functioning objectively as the detached observer, it can offer a very important perspective—one that will take you away from the burden of the subjective interpretation of your sensations that is associated with chronic pain. The ability to perceive from the *I* as the objective observer is an important function of the mind's ability to achieve nonjudgmental awareness of oneself. This may sound difficult to achieve, but with practice, using disciplines—such as the exercises in this book—it is possible.

I is also the *agent.* This *I* is able to make mental representations of perceptions using the cognitive abilities of the cerebral cortex that give the self the objective information necessary for knowing what it intends to do in the world. *I* also uses these cognitive abilities to enable the self to act on these intentions through goal-directed behaviors and make them happen. When the *I* enables the self to accomplish these intentional acts in the world, a person is said to have *agency.* Agency is a sense that the *I* has about how much ability one has to accomplish things in the world. The *I* that has a high sense of agency is able to accomplish much in the world. However, when the *I* identifies too much with the subjective interpretations of the *Me*-self, its cognitive ability to make accurate mental representations of its perceptions is diminished as is its potential for agency. *This is how agency is dramatically compromised by chronic pain, and for healing to take place, agency must be reclaimed.*

The *I* as objective self and the *Me* as subjective self are important perspectives that the mind has the ability to take. It will be crucial, as we continue, that you have a clear understanding of what these concepts mean, as they will be central to your ability to overcome chronic pain.

More about the autobiographical narrative

As we have noted, the autobiographical narrative is the story of one-self maintained in memory. If you were to sit down and write the story of your life, it would be your autobiographical narrative. The autobio-graphical narrative not only influences who you think you are, but it also influences what you are thinking about now and how you process present information. The autobiographical narrative is an important part of the mind, for it creates a sense of who one is and a sense of what importance one may have as an individual, as a member of a group, or as a member of something larger than the self. As we continue in the book, I will often refer to this narrative because the autobiographical narrative of people with chronic pain is very much couched in suffering.

The autobiographical narrative is continually updated as you move forward in the world. Your *working memory,* described earlier, allows you to process present information and arrange that information into a mean-ingful narrative that fits with your autobiographical narrative. This gives your life some sense of order.

However, just as a computer has programs that it follows, your mind has a program. Scientists' understanding of this program is limited at this point. We believe the mind's "program" must be somehow connected with the meanings (memories) we have stored in our mind and somehow connected with the things we see in the world. Our program must fol-low rules, just as our written and spoken language has rules of grammar and syntax that allow us to put that language into meaningful sequences. The program guides the mind's ability to process information, so that it can perceive, remember, and synthesize information in the present with events and experiences we remember. This enables the mind to take pres-ent and remembered information, and put it into some new format so we can make plans for the future and create new ideas.

Psychologists use the word *schema* to describe the programs that the mind uses in order to process information. In a way, they are like the pro-gramming that a computer uses. That is, there are certain rules that allow us to process information and arrange it into a meaningful narrative.

As we continue, it will be important that you realize that your schemas have been dramatically altered by chronic pain and any past events, such as trauma or physical injury (as discussed in earlier chapters), that have led you to be susceptible to the development of chronic pain.

Conclusion

I realize this may have been a difficult chapter to follow. Scientists and philosophers are still learning about the mind, its rules, and its programming. But we do understand aspects of how the mind works, and your knowledge of this information will help you clear yourself of chronic pain. Here are the key points to remember:

1. *Mind* is the part of us that takes our perceptions of the external environment and internal body and puts them into a story that helps us make sense of ourselves in the world.

2. *Meaning* refers to the way we interpret what we experience, perceive, or imagine. There is a correspondence between what we perceive and what exists in the world, and we are able to perceive things in both the internal world (in ourselves) and the external world.

3. *Perception* is the act of receiving stimuli from external or internal sources, also called *sensations.* Sensations include those of sight, sound, touch, taste, and smell. Individual sensations are composed of *qualia,* the elemental properties of sensations that exist in your body.

4. The mind has access to things from the past that we remember in different forms of *memory:* working memory (used from moment to moment), semantic memory (the memory of meanings), episodic memory (the memory of specific events), and autobiographical memory (the memory of our personal history).

5. *Attention* is the capacity of the mind to select and prioritize certain aspects of the environment. The mind has the ability to place attention on important aspects of the environment, recall information from stored memory, and process information so that the world has meaning.

6. *Awareness* (in this book) refers to the skill of perceiving internal and external events without interpreting or judging them. It includes *self-referential awareness,* which is the remarkable capacity to be aware of the self as an *I* that perceives and acts *and* as a *Me* that has a self-image, a history, and other unique features. The mind also has the ability to perceive from both the *I* and the *Me* self-referential perspectives.

7. Finally, the mind uses all of the previous qualities as it creates an *autobiographical narrative*—the ongoing story of your life that is your sense of who you are. The mind uses its capacities to perceive, assemble meanings, retrieve memories, and be aware as it constructs and stores the ongoing autobiographical narrative in the context of the past and the present.

In this chapter, I noted that specific parts of the mind were changed by chronic pain, such as your capacity to be an agent in the world, your sense of who you are, and your ongoing narrative. The next chapter will further explore how these aspects of mind have been changed by pain and how different aspects of mind that are captured by pain can be overcome through exercises, such as the ones in part 2 of this book. As noted, the aspect of mind called awareness will be key to clearing yourself of the burden of chronic pain.

• • •

8

The Mind and Chronic Pain

In the last chapter, we discussed the concept of mind and examined all of the complexities that appear when we attempt to understand it. We were able to break mind down into some of its important components, such as perception, meaning, and memory, to name a few. This was a lot of information to take in, and much of it was likely new to you, so don't worry if you do not completely understand everything that was covered. Take time to think about what you read and especially how these ideas have played out in your life. It may help to review the chapter conclusions, which provide a good reference point for remembering the major points and definitions of each chapter, as you proceed through the rest of the book. In this chapter, I will review the components of mind that we discussed and explain how they have been changed by pain, and then discuss examples of people whom I have seen and treated to demonstrate how pain can impact a person's life. My hope is that these examples will help you recognize how you (or a loved one) have been changed by pain.

We have just explored the mind's ability to represent information and give us an ongoing narrative of how this information has meaning. In a metaphorical sense, it is almost as though there is a movie playing in our head at all times. This movie is the way that the mind is representing the world before you, the world inside of you, and what you are thinking about that world. From this perspective, it should be easy to imagine that what is being projected onto the movie screen has something to do with not only what you are thinking about presently, but also what you have experienced in the past.

Your movie has a theme that goes back as far as you can remember and is even influenced by things that you cannot remember. If you were to use it to make a timeline from birth, you would be able to come up with a story of your life. That is the best way I can describe *autobiographical narrative,* a concept I introduced in the last chapter. It is the story of your life that you have stored in your memory, but it is also the story of what you are experiencing in the present. It influences who you think you are, who you think you can be, and how you refer to yourself. Recall that in the last chapter, I explained that how you refer to yourself is the *Me* of self-referential awareness. So, as we continue, remember that chronic pain has dramatically influenced your autobiographical narrative. It also has had significant influence on the *Me* of that narrative. Most of this influence involves things that have been taken away from you as a result of having chronic pain and not being able to accomplish the things that you used to be able to do. Let's take a closer look at how chronic pain influences all aspects of the mind. As we proceed, I hope you will consider how these influences apply to your life and experience, and begin to gain a new perspective.

Perception and Attention

I, the perceiver, is able to be conscious of the world. *I*-the-perceiver is able to choose those aspects of the world that are deemed important and put attention toward them, *even before any interpretation of these aspects of the world has occurred.* That is, even before the autobiographical narrative lends interpretation to your life.

Chronic pain changes the *I*. *I*-the-perceiver no longer has the ability to put attention on what it needs to attend to for optimal well-being. Instead, attention has been hijacked by the *Me* aspect of self that interprets internal sensations in terms of the autobiographical narrative. With trauma and other adverse events from the past coloring this narrative, the *I's* attention is under the influence of chronic pain. When that attention is under the influence of chronic pain, it is attracted to negative aspects of the world, and even benign aspects are more likely to be perceived as threats. The mind in chronic pain dramatically skews perception and puts great value and attention on things that are perceived as a threat. Let's look at an example of how this may work.

"J." has chronic lower back pain. She is simply interested in rising from bed after poor sleep and going outside for a walk first thing in the morning. When she begins getting up from bed, her attention is captured by the sensation of pain and all of the negative things that it means to her, as her autobiographical narrative has influenced her *Me*-self's interpretation of present events and sensations. All of the other aspects of the world that she wants to attend to are no longer the focus of her attention. Her attention is captured by the threat that chronic pain presents to her. J., as *I*-the-perceiver, is significantly altered. Her attention and perception are captured by pain. As time goes by, this continues to have a dramatic effect on her ongoing autobiographical narrative. As we continue to follow J.'s story, you will see that much more than just *I*-the-perceiver has been altered.

Meaning

You will remember that the mind interprets the world and gives it meaning so that a person (the self) has an understanding of what is going on in the present and knows what to expect in the near future. These meanings correspond with what the self has learned to be true of the world. In the last chapter, we used the example of the different meanings that can be attached to a chair—for example, a thing to sit on and rest or to stand on to change a lightbulb. It is necessary that meanings have continuity and consistency throughout our lifetime. From one day to another, there is a consistency to the meaning of the chair.

As we have seen, chronic pain can dramatically alter our interpretation of the world, the meaning we attach to the world, and even the objects we see in the world. Let's continue with J.'s story as an example.

Prior to experiencing chronic pain, J. had been an accomplished tennis player. She looks at her tennis racket after she rises from bed and starts to realize that she may not even be able to take the walk that she wanted to because of the pain, much less play tennis. She also realizes that the tennis racket no longer has the meaning it once had and has taken on a much different meaning as a result of her chronic pain. She cannot conceive of herself realizing her dream of going out on the court and being a competent player or teaching her grand-children how to play tennis. The tennis racket now carries the meaning of "a person who is no longer able to play tennis." She is no longer competent and will never be able to share the skills she developed over the years with the people she cares about. The meaning of the tennis racket is now one of broken dreams, failures, and a body and mind that is no longer able to produce what it once could. This meaning spreads across all of her life, and she now feels inadequate as a person, partner, spouse, and grandparent. Chronic pain has brought negative meanings to most aspects of J.'s life.

As you can see, the changes in meaning for J. have created a mind that is primed for a future of more pain, as it is clouded by her negative thoughts and emotions. The pain J. is experiencing extends well beyond the pain in her back. It is now a pain that has dramatically changed her life and makes her feel inadequate and no longer the person she once was. The changes in the meaning of J.'s life are predicting a future that is guaranteed to include more pain.

Memory

As I explained in the last chapter, memory is defined as the brain's ability to store information and to recall that information when needed. We have also learned that the ability to recall and to use present information is negatively affected by chronic pain.

As you may remember, *working memory* is the memory we use from moment to moment to bring order to our world. Chronic pain is a great source of interference that has a powerful effect on working memory. Ideally, working memory should be under the control of the individual who is using it to make sense of the world and accomplish goal-directed behavior. However, the person with chronic pain experiences constant interference from the signal of chronic pain and all of the negative emotions and memories associated with it.

Some of you may remember using old radios that had a dial to locate and fine-tune an AM station. If we could not direct the dial to the exact point where the station signal was, the station would come through with a large amount of static. If we were directly tuned in to the station, there was no static and we could hear the voices or music clearly. When working memory is functioning properly, it is like a fine-tuned radio station; the dial is set perfectly to the station and there is no static interference. When one is in chronic pain, there is more interference—an increase in static. This interference comes in the form of the "signal" of pain and all of the associated burden and suffering. Let's continue with J.'s story.

> J. has decided against taking a walk this morning because her lower back pain has been overwhelming. She has decided instead to read a book. However, when she sits down to read, she cannot get through one page. She does not remember what she has read, and she is not able to keep her attention on the words because of the recurrent intrusions of the pain and thoughts of how bad it is making her feel.

You may recall that *semantic memory* is the memory that allows us to store meanings and apply those meanings to what we are thinking about. We have used the example above of how J.'s world has taken on new meanings dictated by her chronic pain. This is common in people who have chronic pain. The meaning of their world has changed dramatically, and they often say that pain has taken away any positive meaning that their lives once held.

Episodic memory is the ability to recall specific events that have happened in one's life. For an example, let's turn again to J's story.

> J. has the ability to recall that she was once a competent tennis player. She recalls that she was all-conference in college and was able to achieve the conference championship as the number two player on her team in her senior year. Until the onset of chronic pain, J. was extremely proud of these accomplishments, but today the episodic memory of her being handed the trophy as the conference champion only brings on sorrow. This is because chronic pain has caused her to believe that she can

no longer be that person who is able to play tennis and enjoy it. *It is almost as though chronic pain has gotten inside of her and changed the memory that once brought her joy into one of regret and sorrow.*

Autobiographical memory is the collective memories that give us the story of our lives.

We have given many examples of J.'s experience that show how her autobiographical memory has been altered. She now sees herself as a hollow person and all her memories of what she once was are overshadowed by what she perceives herself to be now. J. often wonders whether her current life holds any meaning and whether it is worthwhile for her to continue on this earth.

Such thoughts are all too common in people who have endured chronic pain for extended periods of time. Probably worse is that they see themselves as having no productive future.

As can be seen from the above example, chronic pain has a marked effect on memory and can even alter memory or change the emotions associated with certain memories from positive to negative. Chronic pain also generally impairs people's ability to recall information from memory. This can be rectified with practice, and many aspects of memory can be improved.

Self-Referential Awareness

In the previous chapter, we described self-referential awareness as the *I* and the *Me* perspectives. The *I*-self has two jobs: (1) to perceive neutrally (without judgment) external and internal events and sensations, and (2) to take action or have *agency*. We have described above how the *I* perspective can be altered with chronic pain. The things we perceive are changed as attention is manipulated and controlled by the *Me*-self's experience of chronic pain.

You may recall that the *Me* of the referential perspective gives you an idea of who you are. The *Me*-self is the seat of our self-image. It is how we perceive ourselves or the self-concept we have. We have reviewed some examples of how J.'s self-concept has changed dramatically. She has lost her sense of agency (the action job of the *I*-self) and her *I*-self is seen as no longer able to accomplish many things in the world because it has identified with the negative narrative of the *Me*-self that perpetuates her pain. When this is compared to the competent, active self she remembers being, it causes grief and sorrow, which only generates more negative thoughts, and these, in turn, feed J.'s emotional hurt to create more pain.

Chronic pain causes a dramatic weakening of one's self-concept. Like J., people in chronic pain often perceive themselves as inadequate, as no longer productive members of the family, society, or world as they become less and less active. Interestingly, experimental work has shown that chronic pain sufferers often have an incorrect perception of how much they move. In chapter 2, I pointed out that when chronic pain patients are asked how much they move during the day, they report having moved very little and believe that activity or movement will cause them pain. However, when they are objectively assessed and followed to verify how much they actually move, they are often found to have moved nearly as much as a person without chronic pain. This points to a profound mismatch in what chronic pain patients perceive and what actually occurs. *Their self-referential abilities and sense of agency have been dramatically altered.*

Autobiographical Narrative

We have talked quite a bit about the autobiographical narrative; however, it is important to reiterate that in people with chronic pain, the autobiographical narrative is continually being informed by the negative thoughts and emotions that their chronic pain generates and that in turn perpetuate the pain. It is almost as though the author of the autobiographical narrative is continually rewriting the story and leaving out any thoughts of hope or positive change. The good news is that no matter how dark and sad the story of people with chronic pain becomes, it can be "rewritten" for the better.

Information processing

You may remember in the previous chapter that we described the mind as having the ability to continually process information, store information, and come up with a narrative that helps us understand the world. We stated that the mind has *schemas,* or rules for processing information, much like a computer has programs. Chronic pain dramatically alters one's schemas, in that people in chronic pain feel as though they are no longer capable and lack the ability to have an active and meaningful life again. The schemas of people with chronic pain are shunted toward negative emotions and thoughts that may have been set in place long before the onset of chronic pain. It is almost as though one has taken on a negative view of the world fueled by the running commentary *I cannot do . . .* and *I will never be able to accomplish . . .* Analyzing the schemas that we use to process our world will become an important aspect of recovery from chronic pain as we progress in this book.

Awareness

In chapter 7, we described *awareness* as the ability to simply be present. Many of the exercises in part 2, including the breathing exercise introduced in the next chapter, will help you use *mindfulness* techniques to develop awareness in this sense. It is the ability of the *I* to perceive without interpretation of external and internal experiences. This is an ability that people with chronic pain do not have. Several times I have used the analogy of a movie that is constantly running on a screen in your head. Consider for a moment what would occur in your mind if the movie was turned off and the screen was blank. Would there be judgment? Would there be suffering? If J. turned off her "movie," would she interpret her world in the same way as when her schemas are being controlled by the thoughts and emotions associated with her chronic pain?

Consider that being able to appreciate simple awareness might mean experiencing relief from the burden of negative judgments and interpretation that is imposed by chronic pain. What would it mean for J. if she *could* turn off her movie, her interpretations of pain? What would it mean for you?

Conclusion

If you are experiencing chronic pain, it likely has had a significant negative effect on how your mind experiences and interprets the world. It is now important to start asking if you have allowed chronic pain to take over your life because you think (or have been told) that there is no way out—no alternatives to feeling pain. This is a passive approach. I challenge you to begin to think that, indeed, there *is* a way out and it may be much less difficult than you imagine. In the next chapter, we will continue our exploration of the mind and talk about three different types of mind: intellectual, emotional, and the overself—the seat of awareness.

• • •

9

Three Minds

Now it is time to analyze the mind in a different way. I have chosen to do this using a method that will help you understand some of the exercises that will come later in the book.

Most of us would agree that every thought has a theme or meaning. By this I mean that every thought has a story attached to it—every thought is about something. You may be thinking about your job, you may be thinking about your family, or perhaps you are just daydreaming. When you are doing any of these things, there is a sort of theme or meaning that runs throughout the thought process. In this chapter, I am asking you to imagine that the mind itself has three basic, very broad themes. This categorization is simply to help you understand the chapter and later go on to understand how the mind might work when it is in pain. Although there is no specific scientific evidence that these are the only categories the mind has, these categories have been used for thousands of years to explain how the mind works. They are simply a useful way to describe the mind. Let's begin to look at how this might work.

Imagine that you have just checked into a hotel and need a break, so you pick up the remote control and turn on the TV. It is a small town, and you are not sure what channels are available, so you begin searching.

- You press the remote and turn on channel one. It is the intellectual channel! You have seen this channel and you know it will stimulate your thoughts. From history to math to physics to neuroscience, this channel offers the opportunity to learn new concepts and gain new understanding.

- You press the remote again and switch over to channel two. This is another familiar one, the emotional channel. From depths of despair to peaks of joy to long hours of "mellow," this channel will allow you to experience an astounding array of emotions.

- On a whim, you press the remote again and a new channel pops up. Channel three is not available in your hometown. The third station is different! It is called the *overself* channel. This station somehow magically streams information so that it appears in your mind without the constraints of intellect or emotion. On this channel, information may suddenly appear in your mind that you have never before been aware of. Channel three offers an experience of self-awareness and reflection that does not involve an active mind.

These three channels are really different general themes of how we think or ways that the mind functions. We all have the ability to analyze (the intellectual channel) and we all have the ability to experience emotions (the emotional channel). The third ability, the *overself,* is an ability that you may not be aware of. You may have thought of this capacity as spirit, not in the religious sense but more like the original definition of spirit as "breath" or as a nonmaterial life force. Fortunately, with practice, you can learn to observe the overself mind just as you do with the intellectual mind and the emotional mind.

Picture having these three choices right before you. It becomes necessary to give them some thought and try to understand what each means. One channel will stimulate your ability to think, your intellect. It has the possibility of being quite fulfilling, as it will allow you to consider ideas that you have never thought before. But it can also be limiting because it can be difficult to shut off, or because you may have lost the ability to shut it off completely. The other channel will move both your mind and your body and will fill you with emotional experiences. Some will be happy and some will be sad. You may be able to relate to this channel and realize that you have had identical experiences before, and both happy and sad emotional memories can be recalled. This channel may give you a deeper understanding of what these emotions meant to you. It may help you to put these emotions into more focused context. But it will give you little insight into who you are.

The last channel is somewhat different. Without the more familiar intellectual and emotional aspects of thought, you may at first feel disoriented by what appears and it will not make sense. But if you give it time, this channel will allow you to stop analyzing and to simply perceive as the *I*-self (who you are and how you arrived at the moment in time that you currently exist in). Your mind has these three channels or states: intellect, emotion, and overself (detached observation). In this chapter, I will challenge you to ask yourself which of these channels (minds) you are most comfortable in. Previous chapters have discussed how the intellect and emotions are affected by chronic pain, but now it is time to further explore these different minds and see how they may contribute to what is keeping you in pain.

Though this chapter is short, it contains important information. Please pay close attention to the content and review it again if needed. What I am proposing here is that only by allowing yourself to take the time to periodically put aside the intellectual and emotional minds and identify more with the *I*-self will you be able to overcome chronic pain. It is not as hard as you think; it just takes practice. I challenge you to begin that journey now.

Intellectual Mind

The well-known French philosopher Descartes stated, "I think, therefore I am." This statement assumes that there is a thinker. The ability to think and analyze assumes that there is one who is analyzing. Take a moment to consider, Is the *thinker* the intellectual mind or is it someone else? Let's begin to ponder this unusual question: Just who is doing the thinking? For now, accept on faith that there is someone behind the intellect who is able to perceive. I know it may sound mysterious or confusing, but be patient and go with me on this.

The intellectual mind begins to develop at a very early age. We start to understand what things in the world mean and the relationships we have with the many things in the world. Things we perceive in the world can be objects or they can be people. We also begin to understand that things in the world have a constancy (they do not disappear) and that we can expect certain cause-and-effect relationships to continue. For example, we begin to learn that certain actions will get attention; a certain cry may bring food, and eventually, words may be used to request specific foods. This is the beginning of our intellect. We also begin to develop a relationship with ourselves. At a certain age, generally between two and four, we become aware of ourselves as separate people and begin to analyze our thoughts and behaviors and make evaluations. We begin to realize which thoughts and behaviors succeed in meeting our needs and which ones do not.

As time continues and our intellect matures, we make ever-greater use of our ability to analyze and evaluate. With time and practice—and the guidance of adults and support of peers—we become more and more accurate in our evaluations through the accumulation and analysis of data (that is, information about the world and ourselves). These intellectual evaluations produce a wealth of knowledge that helps us to negotiate our way through life.

As we continue to develop the intellect, we understand more and more about how the people and objects in our world work. We can come to a place where we have gained mastery of many subjects and many concepts. The intellectual mind can help us achieve academic degrees, and it can help us obtain jobs with good monetary benefit. But unfortunately it tells us very little about our inner selves.

The intellectual mind constantly evaluates, analyzes, and compares. These abilities are extraordinarily important in navigating many daily challenges and accomplishing many tasks in life, but in some people these abilities take over and are used in situations where analysis or comparison is not required and in fact can become a liability. This is the case for many people with chronic pain. They constantly analyze and evaluate their sensations and abilities, which usually only brings them more pain—and then they try to analyze and evaluate *that* pain, ad infinitum, so that these behaviors become unremitting. Consider our friend J. from the last chapter, a woman who relentlessly analyzed herself. She would compare the competent person that she remembered herself being with the incompetent person she believed herself to be today. Her self-judgment—her self-analysis—became overwhelmingly harsh as she treated herself without mercy. This is what often occurs when people with chronic pain overuse the intellectual mind. Harsh self-judgment can become automatic so that we come to evaluate our abilities and potential negatively, without thinking, in almost any situation.

You might ask yourself now if this overreliance on the intellectual mind fits you. Does your self-analysis regularly take you to a place of harsh self-evaluation? Like J., do you analyze until the analysis becomes self-defeating? Do you come up with helpful answers to your pain by using your intellectual mind, or has the intellectual mind itself become a painful place for you to be? Do you feel trapped and unable to escape from it?

When we think of some of the important discoveries that have been made in our world, such as cures for diseases and technological advancements, we generally believe that they have come about as a result of the intellectual mind. I believe, however, that when people come up with a new idea, they have gone beyond the intellectual mind to a creative place in themselves that is just as important to their discoveries as their intellect. Is it possible that when someone has an "aha" experience, that such a so-called stroke of genius comes about because the person has learned to master the intellectual mind and has gone to a place where natural creativity is allowed free reign?

Ask yourself now if you think it is possible to shut the intellectual mind off. Are there times when you do not analyze and allow yourself to have a quiet mind? Is there another part of yourself behind the intellectual mind that is able to watch its workings with detachment? Are you able to access that part of yourself and release yourself from the control of the intellectual mind?

The intellect can become a continuous progression of perceptions, thoughts, and concepts that hold one hostage. But there is another aspect of mind or self beyond the intellectual mind. That part of your self has the ability to identify as the *I*-self that we met in chapter 7, the self that can simply perceive the workings of the intellectual mind without comment or interpretation. *I*-the-perceiver has the ability to simply observe the self without becoming entrapped in the endless and fruitless comparisons and evaluations of the intellect. This can be a place of calm and peace, a state of *awareness* that leads to healing.

Emotional Mind

Throughout our lives we experience a myriad of emotions. Emotional experiences have physical, cognitive, and behavioral components that together make up the emotional mind. Some emotions, such as happiness, joy, serenity, and excitement, can be pleasurable and uplifting while others, such as anger, resentment, and shame, can be devastating and leave us downtrodden. Emotions can arouse us and our nervous system in both helpful and not-so-helpful ways and often unpredictably so. The emotional mind is seldom stable and is usually in a state of flux.

Over the years, many psychologists and researchers have come to realize that there is a cognitive component to emotions. That is, the emotional mind involves thinking that is different from what occurs in the intellectual mind. Thoughts associated with emotions, generally, have a narrative. There is also a somatic (body) component. Some sensations that accompany emotions can be felt inside of our body, so emotions are complex in how they are experienced. They are not only felt in the body (such as the painful feeling in our chest when we lose a loved one, a pain that inspired the term "broken heart"), but they are also experienced in the autobiographical narrative (such as, I am now the tragic, grief-stricken person who was betrayed by a loved one), and they are felt directly (the sadness, anger, and shame that can result from the betrayal that causes a broken heart).

Scholars disagree about which comes first: the cognitive (thinking or narrative) component or the somatic (body) component. Some have argued that the first to be experienced is the cognitive component. Others have argued that emotions are first felt in the body and then the cognitive component appears. Recent studies have shown that they probably occur simultaneously, although the cognitive component may, at first, remain unconscious. Whatever the final answer may be, the emotional mind has the ability both to be very helpful and to get us into a large amount of trouble. While ideally emotions would be under the control of the perceiver, at certain times, emotions seem to rule us and dictate what we experience. Emotions can be accompanied by moments of great passion, and sometimes these moments gain hold of us and take command of our actions. One thing is for sure: emotions are dependent on a person's ability to perceive them and interpret them. So, as was the case with the intellectual mind, there must be a "thinker" behind the emotional mind.

To better define emotions, think of emotions as landing somewhere on a line (a continuum) that you have drawn in front of you. On one end of the line is the most positive emotional state, the best high or feeling of elation that you could experience. This is the end of the line where positive emotions reside. On the other end of the line lie the most painful emotions, for example, feelings of grief or shame so deep as to create a hopeless state. This line defines the two poles of emotions, positive and negative. Psychologists and cognitive neuroscientists talk about the concept of *valence*. An emotion's valence is its value on the continuum from very positive to very negative. Each emotion you experience has a valence. States such as chronic pain dramatically alter the valence of emotions and have strong control over the emotional mind.

Let's consider J.'s emotional mind.

> As we discussed in the previous chapter, J. spent time thinking about how she had changed as a result of chronic pain and how chronic pain had taken so much away from her life. She began to spend more and more time in the emotional mind, and her emotions mostly fell on the extreme negative end of the emotions continuum. Interestingly, the more J. experienced these negative emotions, the more she would experience pain. And the more she experienced pain, the more negative emotions would come. She was caught in a very vicious cycle. As we stated earlier, this had nothing to do with any physical injury that she had. Most of her pain was being created by emotions. Simply feeling negative emotions in the body made more and more pain for J.

An important lesson to learn is how to escape from the emotional mind, because it has the potential to hold you hostage. This is especially true when the emotions being experienced are slanted toward the negative side. Are you aware of being in your emotional mind much of the time? Can you identify the feelings and thoughts that are attached to these emotions? Begin to watch and recognize how much time you spend in the emotional mind. Is it helpful or is it working against you? Are most of your emotions leaning in the positive or negative area of the emotions continuum? If they are mostly in the negative area, do you recall a time when your emotions were more varied or even mostly positive? If so, can you make the connection between your movement toward more negative emotions and when you began to experience chronic pain?

Overself Mind

We posed the question, Is there a thinker who exists behind both the intellectual and the emotional minds? Let's take a look at what that thinker may look like and if it is possible for such a thinker to detach itself from both the emotional and intellectual minds and avoid being "captured" by them. I am suggesting that there should be a place where this thinker can exist that is quiet and free from evaluation and judgment, a place where it is not at the mercy of emotions and is able to process information from the intellectual and emotional minds without judging or evaluating it. You can know this place best by actually *experiencing* it, since this overself mind, by definition, does not lend itself to intellectual description. However, I will try to give you a glimpse of what that experience might look like as background to the mindfulness exercises in part 2 and the breathing exercise just ahead in this chapter that help one achieve *awareness,* or what I also call a *quiet mind.*

The overself exists behind both the intellectual and the emotional minds, and when one is in the overself, the whole mind is quiet and there is no analysis, evaluation, or judgment—only unhindered observation of the self as it is. It is where the pure knowledge of self—beyond the linear, cause-and-effect thinking of the intellectual mind or the unpredictable workings of the emotional mind—lies. This is the kind of knowledge that comes from direct awareness of the self and makes it possible to really understand and accept who you are. What would have happened to J. if she were able to get access to her overself? Since the overself does not judge and does not hold on to emotion, at least for the time she was inhabiting her overself, J. would have found some respite from the harsh self-judgment and analysis that kept her trapped in a cycle of emotional negativity. She may have been able to see how her chronic pain had resulted largely from being locked in the negative feedback loop created by her intellectual and emotional minds.

A simple exercise: Breathing

Mindfulness meditation is an adaptation of Buddhist meditation practices in which practitioners learn to be mindful—the intentional, accepting, and nonjudgmental focus of one's attention on the emotions, thoughts, and sensations occurring in the present moment. I want to finish this chapter with a simple exercise, based on mindfulness meditation techniques that I encourage you to practice every day. This exercise will be repeated in part 2 as the foundation for the other exercises designed to help you develop mindfulness.

Within days of beginning this practice, many of my patients report getting glimpses of the overself I described above. You will know you are there when your mind becomes simply quiet. You will feel a sense of peace that you may have never felt before and that you will want to experience more and more. And with daily practice, this can happen.

BREATHING EXERCISE

Close your eyes, sit up straight in a chair with your feet on the floor, and place your hands in a comfortable position. Try to maintain a straight back with your hips positioned in a way that they are supporting your spine. If you are unable to attain this position, just try to assume the most comfortable position you can. Now, with your eyes still closed, notice if your mind is quiet or if it is just running on its own. If it is running on its own, it may be the intellectual mind (where your analytical, evaluative thoughts dominate) or the emotional mind (where your thoughts about your emotional states dominate) at work. Now place your attention on your breath, first on the inhale as the air goes through your nostrils, noticing how it feels for air to slowly move into your nostrils and pass all the way into your lungs, and then on the exhale as the air is released into the atmosphere. As you continue placing your attention on your breath, actively slow your breathing down. Try to achieve about six to eight breaths per minute if you are able. Just do your best and be sure that you remain comfortable. Do not let the focus of counting breaths distract you from the goal. You will begin to notice that by simply slowing your breathing,

CONTINUED

you will start to relax and you will be able to watch your thoughts and feelings with more detachment. Eventually, with practice, your mind will start to quiet and you will begin to drift into the part of your mind I have called the overself, a state of pure observation without judgment of the thoughts passing through your awareness. Something this simple will begin to give you some sense of relief. Try to make the time taken for your inhalation the same as the time taken for your exhalation. Hold the breath for just a split second between your inhalation and your exhalation. *Practice this for ten to fifteen minutes twice a day if possible, or at least as often as you can.*

You might also begin to notice how much time you spend in the intellectual mind or in the emotional mind throughout the day and pay attention to whether they are under your control or whether they just function automatically. See if you are able to shut them off at the end of the day or at different times during the day or if they appear to be dominating your consciousness and are outside your control. Among people with chronic pain, these states are generally out of personal control. We will be exploring ways to help you gain more control over these parts of your mind in future chapters and with the exercises in part 2.

Conclusion

In this chapter, you have learned about "three minds": the intellectual mind, the emotional mind, and the overself, the perceiver behind these other states. I likened this to a television with three channels. We have learned that the intellectual and emotional minds of people with chronic pain can bring them to experience very difficult thoughts and emotions. I have asked you to spend some time considering whether you are living more in the emotional mind or intellectual mind, and I have given you a sense of what the third channel, the overself mind, looks like. This channel is one that observes and experiences without passing evaluation or judgment. I have asked you to practice an exercise that will help you enter into the overself, the place where you begin to free yourself from pain and gain a renewed sense of confidence that you do not deserve to carry the burden of pain and suffering.

In the next chapter, you will learn more about the autobiographical narrative, including how the intellectual and emotional minds have influenced this narrative so that it plays a key role in sustaining chronic pain.

• • •

10

Autobiographical Narrative

In previous chapters, I introduced the term *autobiographical narrative*. In this chapter, we will gain a deeper understanding of this important concept. As you may recall, autobiographical narrative is the story that you tell yourself about who you are, built out of the cumulative memories of your past experiences. It is an ongoing and unfolding story about yourself that can influence present and future thoughts about who you are. If you thought back as far as you can and then wrote the story of your life, that would be your autobiographical narrative. People with chronic pain have usually experienced adversity in their lives that has profoundly altered their autobiographical narrative so that it no longer accurately reflects what they have been through and experienced. Many times their narrative is limited and controlled by experiences and memories of both physical and emotional pain that create a vicious cycle of increased pain and stress.

The autobiographical narrative serves an important role in determining the content of your present thinking and how you view and evaluate yourself. It is almost as though your autobiographical narrative determines the very kinds of things you are able to think about. Imagine looking at the movie of your life through a lens that is out of focus. The lens places constraints on what you think, and those constraints are strengthened by pain and the unpleasant feelings and thoughts associated with pain.

In the same way, chronic pain has a significant negative influence on the autobiographical narrative. Many people in chronic pain believe they have permanently lost abilities, skills, and potential, and this feeds recurring negative emotions and thoughts that seem inescapable. These thoughts further limit what people believe they can do, and it is as though chronic pain has put the person in shackles. The result is that people with chronic pain often do not exercise and they lose the curiosity to learn and explore new things. *Their autobiographical narrative reflects this negativity and hopelessness.*

Fortunately, you can practice methods that help you look at your autobiographical narrative and begin to understand some of its important aspects. Such practice will help you begin to realize how to release the burden that keeps you in pain. These practices will also help you appreciate how your autobiographical narrative developed and what role it continues to play in your life.

In this chapter, I will provide some questions you can begin to ask yourself to help change your autobiographical narrative. I will also explain why these questions are relevant and how they will help you modify your narrative. I will offer a number of examples derived from my experience treating people with chronic pain, some of whom have been introduced in previous chapters (with names omitted and circumstances changed to protect their privacy). These examples will demonstrate how one's autobiographical narrative can become significantly changed and confined and will help you understand how you can begin to change your own autobiographical narrative.

Framing, Reframing, and Reinterpretation

As we have discussed previously, every thought has a meaning and every string of thoughts has a narrative or story line (see especially chapters 5 and 7). This occurs because the job of our mind is to explain the world. The mind does this by interpreting data and then giving the interpretation a meaning, which is called framing. When we are able to explain and understand the world, we feel safe; and when we feel safe, there is much less stress and fear in our world. If you recall times in your life when you were unable to understand and explain things that were happening, you will probably remember these times as being incredibly stressful.

The brain and mind remember virtually every event that has ever been experienced in one's lifetime. Although we may not have immediate access to all of these memories, they are nonetheless influencing what we think about and how we craft our autobiographical narrative—our means of explaining our place in the world. This is because past experience influences how we process present data. You may recall that schemas are the rules by which the mind processes information. At any given time, schemas are being used to interpret data or information. That interpretation is then framed or given a meaning.

One way of thinking about how the mind explains the present world is to imagine each thought as a picture. The artist or the photographer chooses a scene to capture or interpret, and then that image is framed. That frame surrounds the picture or photograph and gives the image its own sense of completeness and meaning. The type of frame also influences the way we think about the photo and what the photo represents to us—its meaning.

The process of framing a picture is a useful analogy when we consider how the mind gives meaning to the world. Each situation that we experience is perceived. Then the mind interprets the information and gives it a *frame*. That framing of the experience gives it a certain interpretation or meaning, just as the framing of the photograph anchors the meaning of the photo. In each moment that goes by, we are perceiving, interpreting, and framing situations so that we can understand the world.

There are really several steps to this: An event happens to us. We interpret it and give it a meaning, which creates a frame about the event. That frame keeps the meaning in place, just as a picture frame holds the photo in place. It also means that when similar or related events happen to us, we are more likely to use the same frame and give a similar meaning to those events.

Let's look at an example.

> "K." grew up a very happy, outgoing person. He developed schemas that interpreted information in the world and framed most every situation as happy and enjoyable. K. had an accident in which he was injured and lost a family member. He developed chronic pain as a result of this unresolved adversity. Now most information is interpreted and framed as painful and unhappy. His schemas that interpret present data are skewed by painful memories, unresolved grief, and present pain.

By reviewing our autobiographical narrative, we can begin to realize how meanings in that narrative have been framed. It then becomes possible to begin what is referred to as *reframing*—the process of formulating alternative explanations or meanings to experiences or events. This term is borrowed from the psychological technique called *cognitive reframing*, where one identifies and disputes irrational or maladaptive thoughts to make it possible to view and experience events, ideas, and emotions in a more productive or positive way. When you reframe, you reinterpret the original information. For example, K. began to realize how to release grief and reinterpret the meaning of his life. Over time, he began to develop a new interpretation and a new frame that prevented him from creating more pain and stress in his life.

Let's look at what this means for chronic pain by returning to the example of J., the onetime college tennis player now living in chronic pain.

> You will remember from the last two chapters that the way J. framed the world had shifted. She had once seen herself as a talented and capable person, but now she sees herself as someone completely controlled by chronic pain. As an example, the tennis racket that had once symbolized competence and success has taken on a new meaning, one of loss and grief. She had interpreted the tennis racket as a symbol of pain, because she had framed her world as one of loss and limitation.
>
> Now suppose that J. used the concept of reframing to reinterpret the meaning of her tennis racket and, for that matter, her life. Imagine that she put the racket in her hand and slowly moved her body in the ways that she used to hit a forehand, backhand, and serve. With time, she may find that she can gradually reestablish these movements, and she may be able to play tennis again. Another strategy for her might be to just imagine those movements so that she would remember what they were like and how they felt. Such simple strategies of reinterpretation can help her to reframe meaning in her life and may give J. the potential to change her life completely. For example, she might discover that the pain in her back was not related to the purported damage. It was simply because she had not used those muscles in so long that they had become weakened, tight, and were in spasm. If she gently began to stretch them, in a short amount of time they may start to return to normal function. While she may not ever return to her for-

mer high level of performance as a tennis player, she may still be able to enjoy the game, teach, coach, or advise—it would be her choice. Reinterpreting information and reframing would give new meaning to the tennis racket—once framed as a symbol of athleticism and confidence, then as a symbol of loss and pain, and again as a symbol of new options and the capacity to overcome adversity.

Such strategies begin to erase the doubt and return optimism to people who have been led to believe by their chronic pain that they cannot accomplish things.

Learning to reframe

Let's begin to explore how reframing and then reinterpreting that new frame might work. Here are a few important questions to consider about your autobiographical narrative.

1. *As you think about your autobiographical narrative, can you remember any events that may have changed the direction of that narrative in any significant way?*

   For most people, significant events throughout their lives have altered their autobiographical narrative. Earlier, I used the example of S., who experienced numerous adverse events, including abuse as a child. She internalized those experiences, creating recurrent memories that greatly influence how she interprets and frames the world. As a result of this influence, S. had a very poor concept of herself. She did not understand why bad things had happened to her. In some sense she had blamed herself, even though from an objective viewpoint, she knew that this did not make any sense. As S. confronted her chronic pain, it was important that she learn to be honest with herself and recognize that her situation was not her fault and that events beyond her control had dramatically changed her. They had helped create an autobiographical narrative in which she would continue to experience pain. S. began to realize that, through no fault of her own, those early events had set the stage for a future life of chronic pain.

2. *Could there have been more than one event, perhaps a series of events, that changed your narrative?*

These events may have built up over time and set the stage for chronic pain through internalization and the accumulation of chronic stress. For example, unlike S., J. had not experienced any significant adverse events as a child. Indeed, her childhood had been happy and normal. However, as an adult she began to take on too much. She was a wife in a very demanding and stressful relationship. She was a mother with not enough time to spend with a child who had special needs. She had a demanding corporate job. Over time, the accumulation of impossible challenges set the stage for chronic pain and a change in her self-concept. While participating in a chronic pain group, J. and the rest of the group set about describing their autobiographical narratives. When J. first began to explore her autobiographical narrative, she had no idea that the accumulation of those stressors could have prepared her mind for chronic pain. She thought that her life was normal, and when she heard the stories of everyone else in her group, she thought that she was much better off than they were. Then, over time, she began to reinterpret and reframe her autobiographical narrative. She realized that it was the accumulation of many events that made her susceptible to developing chronic pain. Indeed, for J. this realization gave her great insight, and she was able to discover many other options to begin the process of recovering from chronic pain.

3. *Can you remember when you first began to experience pain and the impact that pain had on your narrative?*

Most people with chronic pain have little understanding and insight about how negatively the chronic pain has affected their lives. Although they may talk about how pain is preventing them from living full lives or say things like, "This constant pain is ruining my life," many pretend that things are going to eventually improve on their own and that they will not have to do any significant work to bring about that improvement. Oftentimes they will go to physicians who only treat their symptoms with medications or other temporary relief. Many people also fail to acknowledge how bad they feel inside. They use coping strategies such as avoidance. They ignore the narrative and bodily sensations that come with stored emotions, pretending that things will improve or that they can continue to endure. Instead of acknowledging the enormous change to their lives, they pretend that things are not so bad and are going to eventually improve. For example, the first time I met "E." she had been in pain for over forty years.

> E. had not been able to walk normally for twenty-five years. She had a degenerated spine, worsened by surgery, and she had become very depressed. Yet she had little understanding about the degree to which chronic pain (and the treatments that she had undergone for it) had affected her life. She was barely surviving from day to day. To my dismay, she was under the impression that she was tolerating it all quite well. She did not have any idea that she had become merely a ghost of the person she had once been and could be again. As we began to work together, she realized that she was miserable, but more important, she realized that her current strategy to treat her pain was only creating more misery. Once she began to reframe her autobiographical narrative, she gained insight into how much chronic pain was affecting her life. She realized that she was under constant stress and hardly ever relaxed. Her narrative was on autopilot and she experienced mostly negative emotions. She had lost hope and optimism and had no plan for recovery. She began to see that her interpretations of the world were contributing to her pain. This realization sparked a dramatic turnaround. Soon she was able to walk straight and upright for the first time in over twenty-five years, and she began to slowly exercise and regain her strength.

Simple insight, reframing, and reinterpretation can have a dramatic effect on chronic pain.

4. *Being as honest with yourself as possible, can you remember when the pain really began? Was there a time when you realized that you did not feel okay inside—that you may have been holding negative feelings inside of you?*

Many people with chronic pain cannot remember experiencing any significant adverse event when they were a child, teen, or even young adult. In these cases, there may have been many smaller events that did not seem significant, or even seemed normal at the time, but that nevertheless set the stage for chronic pain. Some may not have fit in at school. Others may have had parents who did not have enough time for them and made them feel alone. The experience of "N." provides an example of this.

> N. suffered from chronic headaches and body pain, and he could not recall any significant events in his life that may have set the stage for pain. After considerable time exploring his past, he did recall being held and ridiculed in the back of the school bus by some older boys. N. did not realize the significance of this event at the time, but with further examination he realized that the experience marked the first moment that he did not feel okay about himself, a moment that turned into the negative feeling inside of him that he carried to this day. N. began to reinterpret the gravity that this event held. He even re-experienced the emotions associated with the event and recognized that none of this was his fault or meant that he was a bad person. He realized how this incident had altered his self-concept. Thus, he reinterpreted this event and was able to see his real strengths.

Sometimes, when we cannot recall an adverse event, it is because it is so painful that we have completely repressed it. If you experience strong emotions from recalling a past adverse event, such as sexual or physical abuse, an accident or disaster, or family violence, it is important to seek professional help to work through the trauma. You should consider working with an experienced therapist to deal with any emotions that are revealed and you feel you cannot handle on your own.

I hope these examples help you see how people can use their autobiographical narrative in a positive way to gain insight. I also hope that the questions and examples will help you consider what events have been significant in shaping your own autobiographical narrative. With that knowledge, you can begin to use the tools of reframing and reinterpreting described above to begin to gain insight and change. As you begin to identify the factors or experiences that may have set you up for future pain, these tools will allow you to free yourself from much of the burden that holds you in pain.

Influences on the Autobiographical Narrative

You may remember learning about the concept of the *Me*, or subjective, self in chapter 7. An important part of our subjective self involves our self-concept. Our self-concept strongly influences what our autobiographical narrative will look like and what our schemas will include. For many who have chronic pain, there was a point in time when their self-concept became negative, when their opinion or view of themselves changed and became less self-accepting.

Let's revisit the story of J., the former tennis player.

> J.'s autobiographical narrative changed when she realized that her pain controlled her. She identified a point when she first felt that she no longer had control of her body and her life; this was the point at which her autobiographical narrative became painful and negative. She began to experience increasing self-doubt about what she was able to do and who she was as a person. Yet she had little knowledge that her changed autobiographical narrative—her changed self-concept—was likely the very thing that was keeping her in pain. Her autobiographical narrative was no longer in her hands; it was in the hands of chronic pain. She got to a point where she could no longer escape the negative thoughts playing continuously in her mind. These thoughts created more and more pain for her on levels far beyond physical pain.

Imagine the psychic pain involved in J.'s experience of seeing herself as no longer talented and capable. What would that loss feel like? What would it be like when the symbol of your competence in the world became the symbol of your incapacity?

S.'s negative self-concept developed after experiencing childhood abuse, which set the stage for chronic pain to enter her life. Because she had memories of adverse events stored in both her mind and body, she had created a split between her autobiographical narrative and the emotional experiences she had stored inside her body.

This split occurs when people become wounded by adverse events and learn to cope by ignoring the messages of pain that the body produces. Such a split allows the autobiographical narrative to dominate one's thoughts. The problem with this is that the messages from the body, though ignored, still have a major influence on the autobiographical narrative. The autobiographical narrative becomes fraught with negative emotions, yet the more this occurs the more people try to ignore the messages their body is sending. There is a fear of experiencing these messages although, in reality, most of the pain is being driven by the autobiographical narrative, not by the body messages, which are merely sensations and energy. This also creates a mismatch between expectancy (the fear of pain from the body's messages) and reality (the pain that is actually being created by the narrative).

S. chose to ignore the sensations in her body and put her attention only on the negative narrative. Yet, the stored emotions in her body determined the narrative and made it negatively charged with emotion. This mismatch drove her autobiographical narrative, although she had learned at an early age that the best way to deal with her adversity was to ignore the feelings she held in her body. Such a split only creates more and more adversity and stress, as those memories and feelings continue to drive the direction in which the autobiographical memory can proceed. All of S.'s energy, reserve, and resilience were diverted to maintain this split until she finally reached a point where this no longer worked to distract her from her suffering, and chronic pain entered her body.

Conclusion

The goal of this chapter was to help you understand that your autobiographical narrative can be influenced by experience in ways that can generate stress, and that stress can only serve to create more pain. It is a vicious cycle.

I have explained the concepts of framing, reframing, interpretation, and reinterpretation. I hope that you are able to take the time to review these concepts and put them into practice. Understanding when the burden of a negative autobiographical narrative was framed and where it came from will help you begin to find relief. This will also bring you closer to being able to experience the *overself*—the quiet mind.

The next chapter will provide an overview of stress and what happens when stress becomes chronic. Research is making it more apparent that chronic stress and the inability to turn the stress response off is the problem underlying many chronic illnesses, especially chronic pain. When we come to the exercises in the second part of this book, the ability to shut the stress response off will be a major goal.

• • •

11

Chronic Stress

The human body and the human brain have a mechanism that protects them from actual and perceived threats. This mechanism is called the *stress response*. You may have heard of it by the popular term "fight or flight," which refers to the behaviors that are options when the stress response is activated.

We activate the stress response when we perceive a threat to our well-being. The response involves a number of changes in brain chemistry that prepare us to either defend ourselves or escape. As soon as the stress response begins, other mechanisms in the brain prepare to shut off the response. This is essential because, if the stress response continues for a prolonged period of time, it causes tremendous wear and tear on the brain, mind, and body. Unremitting stress can lead to many diseases, including heart disease, depression, hypertension, and chronic pain. So, if left "on," the stress response stops protecting us and begins to turn against us and damage us.

This chapter will explain what occurs when the stress response is prolonged and becomes chronic. Most people in chronic pain and most people who have experienced significant adverse events have not been able to turn the stress response off for a long time, which is both uncomfortable and unhealthy. After you have finished this chapter, you will be able to apply your newly gained knowledge about the stress response to your life, perhaps to determine if you are under chronic stress and cannot turn the stress response off. If this is the case, then it is important to understand why this has occurred and begin to do the exercises in this book to help regain control of the stress response.

Normal Stress Response

When we perceive a real or potential threat to our well-being, a programmed sequence of events occurs in the body and brain. First, we release a cascade of hormones that result in increased energy, anxiety, and sometimes hostility. These reactions can lead to an often perceptible increase in heart rate and breathing rate, but other changes occur too. Almost immediately, our attention shifts from more thoughtful and contemplative goal-directed thinking to more reflexive responses that enable us to either defend ourselves or flee the situation. Our emotions are aroused, including the emotion and sensation of fear. Simultaneously, our stomach and intestinal processes slow or stop. Our skin often pales or flushes. In many parts of the body, the blood vessels constrict, while in other parts of the body (such as the muscles), the blood vessels expand. In general, vision becomes tunnel-like, focusing on a specific area of the environment—usually where the threat is thought to be located.

Meanwhile, our attention to other areas of the environment is diverted; for example, our pupils dilate in order to take in information. There is generally a freeing up of normally inhibited nerve reflexes, increasing our ability to quickly respond to a threat. We become infused with energy and anxiety and may begin to shake and sweat.

After this initial reaction, the changes in brain chemistry that initiated the stress response quickly diminish and the stress response resolves. All of the above-mentioned physiological responses return to normal or baseline. Our heart and breathing rate slow, anxiety resolves, and normal thinking returns.

Other reactions in the brain, mind, and body

Our stress response also includes an immediate change in behavior and cognition. We become very vigilant and on the lookout for potential threats. We tend to respond to the smallest change in the environment as our attention shifts from goal-directed behavior to a more defensive posture. Our mood often becomes dysphoric or unhappy. Pleasurable experiences no longer bring pleasure, and we do not appreciate the positive feedback that normally occurs with accomplishments.

Our metabolism also changes with the onset of the stress response. Normally, the hormone insulin allows blood sugar (glucose) to be absorbed by body tissues. However, during the stress response, insulin becomes much less effective as the body tries to keep a large supply of energy on hand to fight or take flight. The sympathetic nervous system, a part of the autonomic nervous system that causes the body to become activated and anxious, takes over. Neurotransmitters and hormones, such as cortisol, norepinephrine, and epinephrine, are quickly released, causing us to become highly aware, anxious, and agitated. Our inflammatory response becomes increased, enhancing our ability to clot blood in preparation for possible injury when defending against a predator. The amazing thing is that all of these responses occur automatically as the stress response begins to dominate the brain, mind, and body.

To summarize, when the stress response is activated, the areas of the brain involved in higher-order thinking, planning, contemplation, behavior management, anxiety management, pleasurable reward, and negative emotion management are all inhibited. Meanwhile, areas of the brain, mind, and body that contribute to heightened awareness, surveillance, hypervigilance, anxiety, and increased energy become dominant.

Why would our body have this incredibly unpleasant mechanism? Well, it makes perfect sense and is a healthy short-term reaction to danger. We need to survive an immediate threat. Thinking, pleasure seeking, planning, contemplation, the pursuit of happiness, and digestion do not matter at this point. We need to be breathing quickly with an elevated heart rate to get our muscles well oxygenated, and we want to increase our blood sugar for our muscles, so we can fight or run. We need our inflammatory system ready to go, so if we are wounded our blood will clot quickly. We need to be on high alert for motion or other threats. In fact, when survival is at stake, many normal functions could distract us and make us vulnerable. None of our ancestors would have survived for long if they had stopped to enjoy the beautiful flowers while a panther was rushing at them! The stress response is a magnificent example of our body's response to environmental demand.

If we are truly threatened, the stress response can be lifesaving. However, when the stress response is prolonged, becomes harder to turn off, becomes easier to initiate, or cannot be turned off at all, these responses can become very damaging to the body. Problems begin when more and more aspects of the world are perceived as a threat. For example, there is nothing truly threatening about speaking at a public event, yet for many people this arouses the same stress response as encountering a predator. In our current environment, we face countless sources of perceived threats that are not truly threats to our lives but nevertheless trigger the stress response. When the stress response occurs in situations that are not life-threatening and this becomes a part of everyday life, the result can be very harmful.

Let's see what happens when acute (short-term) stress becomes long-term, chronic stress.

From Acute Stress to Chronic Stress

The stress response can become less regulated or unregulated, and it can become chronic and unmanageable. Research findings suggest that people who are exposed to adverse events at an early age—or at other times throughout their lives—can develop painful emotional memories that increase their risk of developing chronic stress. Some studies suggest this is because the brain and mind prioritize memories according to the threat level that they pose to the individual. So, if you have had many threatening experiences in your life, these memories take priority—that is, the brain accesses and retrieves these threat-related memories more readily than less threatening ones. This makes sense from a survival point of view. Ready access to these memories will help us avoid situations that were previously life threatening (and are therefore likely to be threatening again). The problem seems to occur when those memories of previous threats either predominate or become generalized to other situations. When this occurs, we perceive many things as threatening that do not actually pose a danger at all—such as the "threat" for a battle veteran of being at a Fourth of July celebration where fireworks are set off.

If we experience a high degree of present-day stress and are unable to adequately cope with it, chronic stress may prevail. It is important to note that the cause of our stress can be either external or internal. For example, external stress is caused by something in the environment around us. So, if we are being abused or bullied or threatened, or if we are experiencing repeated physical injuries or illnesses, or if we live in a war zone, a violent neighborhood, a violent family, or other high-risk conditions, these external threats trigger the stress response.

At the same time, we may generate internal stress, as when we ruminate on unresolved painful threatening memories. These memories cause undue anxiety and fear that also trigger the stress response.

In some conditions, the areas of the brain responsible for overseeing the creation of anxiety and stress can become overwhelmed, and the brain loses the capacity to regulate these areas. Then the part of the brain that creates anxiety and fear begins to predominate. Subsequently, the stress response becomes prolonged or constant. It becomes easier and easier to turn on the stress response until it becomes chronic and constant. The stress response has gone from being a normal reaction to a perceived threat that subsides naturally to a chronically active reaction that either does not shut off at all or is increasingly difficult to shut off.

It should be clear that there is no single way that a person transitions from acute stress to chronic stress. Instead, this may happen in many different ways.

- Traumatic events (at any age, but especially during childhood, when the brain is developing) can initiate the stress response. The psychological pain that occurs as a result of painful threatening memories can create a situation of stress that becomes chronic. For example, a child who experiences physical or sexual abuse, serious injury, or neglect might develop an ongoing stress response. An adult who has witnessed or been subject to violence or intense psychological pressure may have a similar response.

- In other instances, a number of stressful events may occur, none of them major, but the accumulation or timing of the events pushes them beyond the individual's coping capacity. Examples might include an athlete who suffers repeated painful physical injuries, a person who has a job that is continually pressure filled and stressful, or a person who is overwhelmed by caring for family members while being the sole provider.

- In other instances, people's expectations for themselves may not match the reality of their lives. Examples might include a person raised to be the "perfect spouse" who enters a difficult marriage, a person who expects to have major financial success but finds it unobtainable, or a person who chooses a career based on parental input instead of one's natural talents and interests.

All of these scenarios (and many others) can lead to a continued and prolonged stress response that becomes unmanageable and chronic. In these cases, professional help may be needed to work through the trauma and come to terms with the repressed feelings that are contributing to the stress.

Homeostasis and allostasis

The body and brain seek to maintain a balanced state. We refer to this as *homeostasis*. The body and brain also have a process that helps them return to a normal, balanced state after experiencing stress. We call this process *allostasis*. Thus when one needs to get up a flight of stairs quickly, the body will adapt by mobilizing energy, increasing heart and respiration rate to deliver more blood and energy to the muscles of the legs and arms so they can move quickly. Once this process has stopped, there are mechanisms in the body that bring it back to a steady state of normal heart rate, respiratory rate, and blood flow.

The stress response is not a balanced state; the body immediately seeks to return to a normal, balanced state after the stress response has been activated. Thus, homeostasis and allostasis are important mechanisms that the body and brain use to adapt to stress and bring themselves back to normal. The more the stress response is called into action, however, the more difficult it is to shut it off, and homeostasis and allostasis become less effective.

Allostatic load

Allostatic load refers to the amount of stress that one has accumulated over a lifetime. The more a person is forced to call the stress response into play to deal with and adapt to threatening physical or psychological situations, the larger the allostatic load one has. To make this clear, I often use the analogy that each of us is born holding a basket. Each time we experience a stressor, a stone gets put in the basket. A larger stressor gets a large stone; a small stressor gets a small stone. As stones accumulate, it becomes harder to hold the basket; the stones can even stretch the basket to the breaking point. When we can no longer hold the basket or the basket breaks, stress becomes chronic—our allostatic load overwhelms homeostasis and allostasis. When stress becomes chronic, all of the stress response mechanisms come into play. Let's review some of them:

- Cognitive skills shift from more goal-directed, thoughtful cognition to more reflexive responses.

- Energy metabolism shifts so that the body does not respond to insulin in the same way and a large amount of glucose is available in the blood. This increases the inflammatory response and can lead to higher instances of blood clotting.

- Heart rate, breathing rate, and blood pressure all increase. This creates a great amount of wear and tear on the brain, mind, and body and is a breeding ground for many chronic diseases.

The brain, mind, and body have a great amount of resilience and are able to use allostasis and homeostasis in the face of many stressful situations. Not everyone is born with the same amount of resilience, though, and some people can endure higher levels of stress than others. Regardless, when we can no longer hold the basket, or the basket breaks, life becomes very difficult as we transition to a state of chronic stress.

Chronic Stress, Chronic Disease, and Chronic Pain

At this point, I suggest you take a moment and review how many stressors you have had in your lifetime. You might begin with your childhood and try to remember if you always felt safe and happy with a good sense of well-being. Then go on to review your adolescence and young adulthood. Now review your present life.

Try to recall when the stressors started. Was it early in life or more recent? Have they been intermittent or steady, and have they continued to increase? Are you presently under a lot of stress? Have you reached a point where you are surviving and just trying to endure life?

When stress becomes chronic, we shift gears from resourceful living to survival mode. Remember, the stress response developed so that we could handle the threats to our lives. In situations where we feel chronically stressed, we are doing no more than trying to survive.

It is not hard to understand why chronic stress can bring on many diseases. Chronic stress affects blood pressure and the cardiovascular system and thus can lead to hypertension, heart attacks, and strokes. Chronic stress also affects the immune system and can make one more likely to develop autoimmune disorders. The compromised immune system also leaves us more prone to contracting viruses or developing bacteria-related illnesses, since our ability to combat these pathogens has been reduced. We also become more susceptible to anxiety, insomnia, negative changes in mood, depression, or depressive-like symptoms. Many recent studies have also shown that chronic stress, combined with genetic, physiologic, and environmental factors, can be a contributing factor to accelerating the aging process. For example, people with chronic stress may experience an earlier-than-normal decline in cognitive abilities.

Sadly, once stress becomes chronic, the vulnerabilities and diseases described above create even more stress for us. This is why I use the term vicious cycle; the added stress of new problems further increases our risk of developing both mental and physical disease, which adds even more stress. 'Round and 'round we go.

Chronic stress also can create chronic pain. Remember, chronic stress opens the door to changes in the brain that put attention on pain (or the threat of potential pain) and take it away from more important goal-directed behavior. It also creates the pathway for all of the problems that accompany chronic pain, such as anxiety, symptoms of depression, and sleep problems such as insomnia.

We learned earlier that the more painful experiences people have had in their lifetime, the more likely they are to develop chronic pain. This is because those pathways in the brain that process painful experiences are the same ones that process any type of pain. While the brain knows the difference between the pain that comes from stepping on a nail and the pain felt from being teased in public, it does not distinguish between physically, emotionally, or socially painful experiences in terms of the stress they cause. In short, all of these trigger the stress response that over time can become chronic. The sensation of pain itself is a very stressful situation that can set off the stress response. When pain becomes prolonged over the course of days, weeks, or months, the accompanying stress can become overwhelming, and if one already has a high allostatic load (a history of adverse, negative, and stressful experiences—a heavy "stress basket"), the possibility of developing chronic pain increases. This is why I have asked you to identify significant stressors in your life, explore whether you are under chronic stress, and if so, determine when that chronic stress response was turned on and whether and when you lost the ability to turn it off.

The good news is that even if your basket of stress stones has gotten too heavy or broken altogether, you can repair the basket and pour out the stones. Some of the exercises I have presented so far, along with your reflections on questions I have asked as we have progressed from chapter to chapter, are already beginning this process. As we continue, you will gain more insight into how to get your stress response back under control.

Conclusion

In this chapter, we have learned about how the stress response functions when it is normal and appropriate and how the stress response works when it becomes chronic. One is adaptive (good) and the other is highly maladaptive, damaging to the brain, mind, and body, and can lead to chronic disease.

I hope that you have gained an understanding of allostatic load and can begin to evaluate how much allostatic load you have now and have had in the past. It is important to recognize which stressors created large amounts of allostatic load in your life. It is also helpful to realize that being in pain chronically creates a very high level of stress and allostatic load in itself. Thus, a vicious cycle develops that includes old painful memories and events, a high degree of present-day stress, and many levels of pain that create more stress. Fortunately, there is another way of approaching life and greatly reducing your allostatic load.

In the next chapter, you will learn more about adversity and its role in chronic pain and stress.

• • •

12

Adversity

In this chapter, we will talk about a term that I have used throughout the book, adversity.

> **Adversity** is defined as any experience or perception that you assess and frame as a threat to your well-being.

This may appear simple, but it is very important that you begin to acknowledge *any* adverse experiences you have had during your life, as they may have had a dramatic effect on how you view the world. More important, the adversity may be causing pain.

Adversity does not have to be an overt threat in the sense that you fear being injured or even killed. It can merely be that a specific experience made you feel a loss of well-being. It may be as simple as experiencing the loss of a friendship or even the feeling of being rejected. Adversity generally has both a negative emotional component and a painful somatic (body) component, although the pain may not be obvious at first. In other words, when you experience or even remember the adverse experience, you may recall, "This made my body feel unwell and it was associated with some form of pain."

As an example, many of us did not feel accepted during our childhood. We may have been provided shelter, food, and security, and this gave us some sense of well-being. Yet on some level, we did not feel completely accepted. Perhaps our parents and family did not quite understand how to make us feel emotionally secure, even though everything else in life seemed okay. This may have created a feeling of a loss of well-being or a sense of emotional pain. The pain was not so bad that it was overwhelming, but over time these negative feelings built up and became trapped as a negative emotional state inside the body. For some children, such an experience may not have a lasting effect, but for others this experience may have changed their future dramatically. So, much of the outcome of adverse experiences depends on how we perceive the experience and how we process the associated emotions and somatic experiences. This means that the experience of not being accepted by a group, family members, parents, or even friends can produce a dramatically different effect, depending on the individual.

Adversity comes in many forms. The sense of not being fully accepted is one common source of adversity that I often hear about from my patients. Others may report that they were doing well as children and then abruptly lost someone close to them. But, no matter what the adverse experience was, the common element is that the individual did not know how to adequately cope with the adversity, and this created a lost sense of well-being—a lingering inner pain.

There are many other examples. For instance, some people are basically anxious and do not feel comfortable around others, or feel as though they do not fit in with any specific group. Some people face challenges stemming from their self-identity or how they are identified by others, such as people who have dealt with discrimination based on their race, religious beliefs, or sexual orientation. For others, adversity comes from being bullied as kids. As adults, some people find adversity when they do not achieve the job status that they wanted or when they have a boss who is overly demanding.

Also, it is important to understand that what is perceived as extraordinarily adverse by one person may not be a source of adversity to someone else. It also does not have to be one "big" adversity; rather, it can be the accumulation of many small adversities. As I stated above, the critical factor is how the specific experiences are perceived and how the associated emotions are processed.

Adversity can be thought of as occurring along a continuum, beginning with very minor situations and ending with extreme, life-threatening experiences. No matter which end of the continuum an experience falls on, any situation or event can be perceived as adversity. Recall that earlier in this book I defined pain as any experience associated with a negative sensation (see chapter 2). With that definition in mind, it becomes clear why adversity is important: adversity usually creates pain and the pain can build up depending on how it is handled. It may be a minor experience of pain, but it counts. If we think of adversity as the opposite of well-being, then we can see that where there is a lack of well-being, there is room for the creation of pain. So, it is important that you recognize where and when in your life you experienced pain from adversity and how you handled it. It is also important that you learn techniques for relieving the burden that you have internalized and for dealing with future adversity in a different way so it will not become internalized (and potentially create even more pain).

As I stated in the introduction to this book, I do not believe humans are created to suffer. I do believe that much of suffering occurs because we are not taught how to process and release adverse events and they become stored as burdens that have the potential to increase our allostatic load and pain. When we have reached a place where this is occurring, the most important thing we can do is identify the adversity that is creating the burden and learn how to eliminate it. The purpose of this chapter will be to help you identify adversity. In subsequent chapters and exercises, you will learn how to relieve the adversity that is creating the burden you have held, sometimes for many years.

Adversity and Chronic Pain

About five years ago my friend and colleague Mark Haviland and I, along with some other colleagues at Loma Linda University Medical School, began to analyze a large data set compiled from a mailed questionnaire about health, lifestyle, and spirituality. The questionnaire had over 10,000 respondents. Our purpose in analyzing this data was to compare people with extremely debilitating chronic pain to a group of people without pain. We wanted to determine what correlates were associated with chronic debilitating pain.

A *correlate* is a factor associated with another factor. For example, hypertension (high blood pressure) is associated with myocardial infarction (heart attack), and tobacco consumption is associated with a number of cancers. In industrialized countries, regular exercise is linked with longevity. This does not necessarily mean that exercise *causes* people to live a long life. Rather, it means that the two factors occur together, and suggests that more research may help us uncover whether the two factors are linked in some way where one causes the other. Researchers might study the relationship between exercise and longevity, and learn that people who live long lives also have a genetic trait that makes them want to be more active. Or they may study the relationship and find out that exercise reduces some other factors that would normally shorten one's life. The important thing here is that when factors are correlated, researchers can do more work to find out how the factors are linked and whether changes in one factor will lead to some desirable change in the other factor.

We used the data set to complete three studies. In our first study we looked at a group of people who a physician had diagnosed with fibromyalgia, a disorder characterized by chronic widespread pain that is often associated with depression, anxiety, and insomnia. We focused on a group of respondents who reported pain that was overwhelmingly debilitating and had a dramatic impact on their quality of life. Our intent was to compare them to a group of people without pain and determine what factors may be associated with this debilitating pain.

Consistently, we found that people with fibromyalgia who reported debilitating pain had experienced significant adversity at some point in their lives. We asked specific questions about physical, sexual, and emotional abuse as well as other stressful events. We also asked whether respondents had experienced a bad accident, or had seen others experience a bad accident. We learned that the people in this subset were also experiencing a very high level of present stress, mostly because of lack of success in life and lack of self-care. They were anxious, had symptoms of depression, did not make good lifestyle choices (did not exercise or eat well, lacked social interaction, and so on), and were not able to get restorative rest and sleep; further, they stated that adverse events in their past were unresolved. The results were striking: over 90 percent reported having experienced significant adverse events during their lifetime. In addition, they reported more co-occurring medical and psychiatric disorders than did the group without fibromyalgia or pain. Our suspicion was that adversity had dramatically changed them at a time when they did not have the coping ability or the resilience to regain a sense of balance in their lives. At this moment, they began to experience chronic stress. However, while our data does not *prove* that this adversity is the cause, it is an important correlated factor to explore.

We approached these results with some caution, because all of the reports of adversity came from memories that had been stored and consolidated for many years and then recalled for the questionnaire. For some respondents, as many as fifty years had passed since the adverse event. Therefore, we knew that some peer reviewers of our research would question the validity of this data that came from self-reports. As a general rule, researchers are cautious when interpreting data that is from self-report—that is, a person recalling information from memory. People may forget, change the memory, be concerned about reporting accurate personal information, and answer the same question differently depending on their emotional state. Still, self-reported data is sometimes the only way to collect information. As someone whose work is primarily about helping people, I generally trust the information that people self-report, but it is important to understand why researchers are cautious about such information.

However, we felt confident that because the report of adversity was so consistent, it would be difficult to discount. It is not completely surprising that people with fibromyalgia would have such a profile, since the diagnosis is still not fully accepted as a medical diagnosis by many in the health care community. Some practitioners still believe that fibromyalgia should be characterized as a psychiatric diagnosis, as there are no definitive medical tests that confirm its existence. Rather, it is a diagnosis of exclusion. This means that after exhaustive medical testing, if no other diagnosis is confirmed, fibromyalgia is often given as a default diagnosis. Many health care providers believe that people with fibromyalgia have a tendency to be overly dramatic. However, I have treated many people with fibromyalgia and I believe that their pain is absolutely real. I also believe that these people are suffering tremendously. Even so, I realize and respect that not all my colleagues agree.

The second study we undertook compared patients with both fibromyalgia and irritable bowel syndrome with a group who had fibromyalgia only, a group who had irritable bowel syndrome only, and a control group with neither condition. (Irritable bowel syndrome is a chronic and common disorder that affects the gastrointestinal system and includes symptoms such as cramping, abdominal pain, gas, diarrhea, or constipation.) The group with both fibromyalgia and irritable bowel syndrome reported similar problems as the group with fibromyalgia only, but the problems they reported were much worse in severity. This suggested another hypothesis to us: perhaps there was an underlying syndrome of chronic stress that preceded and then fueled the chronic pain these people experienced. We hypothesized that this underlying chronic stress could also have fueled the various co-occurring psychiatric and medical problems that were being reported by people with chronic pain. There appeared to be more than just a chronic pain syndrome or a number of chronic pain syndromes that were being reported. What was emerging was an overall report of lack of well-being, high adversity, high present stress, and multiple co-occurring medical and psychiatric disorders. Of course, as we have noted, chronic pain itself can cause a focus on adversity and negative feelings that could partially account for the large number of these kinds of experiences in these reports.

We went on to do the same analysis on all people who reported chronic pain. We included in this study, for example, people who reported lower back pain from degenerative disc disease, people who had headaches, and people who had osteoarthritis with knee and shoulder pain, to name a few. This group had definite medical diagnoses that could be confirmed by radiology, blood testing, and physical exams. We felt that having confirmed diagnoses would give more validity to the data set. We analyzed this group with and without the group of respondents who had fibromyalgia, thinking that the fibromyalgia group may have skewed the data. We were able to confirm that it did not matter what chronic pain diagnosis these people had reported. As many as 90 percent reported significant adverse events. All were under high present stress, and all reported associated factors that were similar to those reported by the group with fibromyalgia and the group with both fibromyalgia and irritable bowel syndrome. They all had multiple co-occurring medical and psychiatric diagnoses, had overall poor quality of life, and were generally unwell.

These three studies helped us develop the idea that major stress experienced during one's lifetime that is framed as threatening (adversity) may be an underlying factor in the development of chronic pain, especially for those who had the most debilitating pain—pain that impacted their quality of life and well-being. There was also a high level of co-occurring medical and psychiatric disorders among this group. Another consideration is whether there is an underlying factor (or several factors) that may account for the development of not only chronic pain but also other co-occurring disorders. Subsequent studies are beginning to support my theory that the underlying factor responsible for chronic stress may be allostatic load (accumulated adversity). This could also account for the high level of present stress. Our studies showed associations among these factors, but subsequent research is beginning to reveal a causal relationship between chronic stress (adversity) and the development of many chronic diseases, including chronic pain. I have been using this idea in my approach to treating people with chronic pain for a number of years.

Adversity in Your Life

Take some time now to review the adversity you have experienced in your life. Ask yourself these questions:
  • How much have you endured?
  • How early in your life did it begin?
  • How much is adversity creating continued stress and
    chronic pain in your present life?

One of the problems most people encounter when they begin to do this work is that they have held adversity for so long that they feel it is just a normal part of life. They do not realize that they carry such a tremendous burden. The burden feels normal to them, so they do not think it is something they should not be experiencing. Most people who come into my program think that their present life is somehow normal, even though they are, for the most part, miserable. They have grown to believe that what they are experiencing is okay. They often compare their own experience with that of others and conclude that although their lives have been bad, they are not as bad as what some others have had to endure. We can always find people who have had it worse than us, but that does not mean our burdens and struggles are not important and should be ignored. This can be one more way we avoid dealing with our pain and hold ourselves in misery unnecessarily.

Try to remember the first time you experienced anything in your life that could have caused you to feel the loss of well-being. This may have been your first painful memory. Remember that adversity is relative to how you frame it and so it does not have to be a life-threatening experience in order to be relevant. Consider those memories that seem connected to pain. Negative experiences that persist in memory are internalized, and this means you may be experiencing the beginnings of chronic pain and not even be aware of it. You should also think about when in your life you began to experience stress and when you realized that your stress had become chronic and out of control.

The questions below can help you explore experiences of stress and adversity in your lifetime.

- Do you often experience anxiety—an uncomfortable agitated feeling inside? This may be related to unresolved issues from the past or the anticipation of adverse events in the future.

- Do you often experience symptoms of depression—feeling sad, feeling inadequate, lacking energy, feeling constantly tired or unable to sleep? For people with chronic pain, this depressed state is generally the feeling that they are unable to accomplish what they should, so there is a large mismatch between actual self and what one feels the self should be.

- Are you your worst critic? Do you judge yourself more harshly than you judge others?

- Are you shy and introverted, often feeling vulnerable, under scrutiny, or alone, even when you are with other people?

- Do you have a tendency to worry and regularly feel as though something is bound to go wrong in the future?

- Have you had experiences in the past that you regret and are still trying to change, if only in your mind by ruminating on them?

These questions are just a few you can ask yourself to begin gaining insight about how you may be creating intrapersonal (internal) stress that is creating a sense of uneasiness and internal pain.

Conclusion

In this chapter, we explored adversity and how adversity can create a sense of uneasiness and chronic stress that will open the door for pain. I have reviewed three research projects that my colleagues and I have conducted. This research has shown that adversity and chronic stress are linked with chronic pain as well as with psychiatric and medical diseases. This suggests that adversity and chronic stress may lead to many psychiatric and medical diseases (although we do not know that for certain). However, this idea opens up useful channels for helping people overcome the burden of chronic pain.

I hope you will begin to consider how much adversity you have experienced and how this adversity may be creating chronic stress in your life. Both adversity and stress seem to be strong contributors to the development and continuation of chronic pain. Many of my patients have entered my program denying that they had serious problems beyond their chronic pain. My observation has been that they release the chronic pain in part by acknowledging the adversities and stresses they have faced, rather than trying to ignore them or make them seem normal.

In the next chapter, we will discuss why people continue to suffer in their lives. As you will see, much of prolonged suffering is caused by the inability to pay attention to a wealth of information contained in your body. This information is often related to adversity that has been internalized and held in our body. In part 2 you will learn specific ways to pay attention to those messages. In the meantime, do not forget to continue to do the breathing exercise I outlined in chapter 9.

. . .

13

Why Do I Suffer?

This chapter will review many of the concepts that have been discussed in the book thus far. Such a review will deepen your understanding of how these factors might impact you and the amount of suffering that you experience.

By now, it should be clear that I believe that chronic pain is first and foremost about suffering. That is, it is not the signal of pain alone that causes suffering. Rather, it is the interpretation of that signal and all of the other things that signal conveys to the person who experiences it. We have covered this concept in previous chapters, but it is now time to apply it to your own experience so you will be prepared to tackle the exercises in the second part of this book.

I do not believe that people are inherently "meant to suffer." I think that the mind, brain, and body have the ability to heal most illnesses and specifically to end the suffering brought on by chronic pain, but in order to do this we must be in balance. This means that part of the job before you is to determine why you suffer. Even if you are experiencing periodic pain but do not have chronic physical pain at this point, you should consider whether you have the potential to develop chronic pain. So let's begin to learn about the process of regaining balance.

In an earlier chapter, I explained that when pain becomes chronic, it is often difficult to establish a clear relationship between the apparent tissue damage in the area where it hurts and the amount and intensity of the person's pain. I also made the case that pain does not have to be in any specific area of the body for it to be present. Indeed, people who are anxious and people who have symptoms of mood disorders may report experiencing a painful feeling in their body.

I have also emphasized the role that adversity plays in the development of pain, and I will remind you that adversity is painful to the body and the mind. Pain does not have to be from a physical injury and can simply arise from a very stressful day or the accumulation of repeated stress over days, months, and years—a large allostatic load. Pain can also be created by the way that one has learned to interpret and frame the world.

This is a short but important chapter that establishes the basis for why the exercises are presented as they are in this book: *they are designed to allow you to change your cognitive, emotional, and spiritual interpretation of the world and, in so doing, regain balance.*

You will note that I have reintroduced the word *spiritual*. Spirituality does not have to be attached to any religion. As I use the term, it is simply the search to be in harmony with the world and any universal force you may believe in that instills in you the optimism to want to heal and the desire to be in balance. I believe that when one is in balance with the world and the universe, there is a healing effect. This healing is spiritual in that it is the result of a natural intelligence possessed by the brain, mind, and body that unifies them as brain-mind-body to create this natural balance or harmony. What I am showing you in this book is simply how to retrain your brain-mind-body and allow this harmony to happen.

Balance

In earlier chapters, I argued that when pain becomes chronic, the mind and brain become unable to function as they should and so suffering occurs. I also pointed out that this is evident in actual structural and functional changes that take place in the brain. (You may remember that important areas of the frontal lobe do not function properly in people with chronic pain.) In the mind, the manifestations are seen with rumination, catastrophic thinking, and the inability to quickly process negative emotions so they have only a minimal lasting effect on health. I also discussed three minds—the intellectual mind, the emotional mind, and the overself. I described the overself mind as the most helpful in the healing process, but stated that because of lack of previous experience with or learning about this part of ourselves or the demands of our current situation, we spend little time in the overself. I talked about how the stress response can become chronic and can increase allostatic load (our "stress basket") to the point where we are overwhelmed, and this diminishes our mental and physical health. Further, I discussed the importance of adverse events in our lives, the importance of how these events are processed, and noted that sometimes adverse events are internalized and kept in our body.

When we gain balance, we are able to do a number of things. First, balance enables us to achieve a quiet mind. A quiet mind, in turn, allows us to access information that is not from the intellectual mind or the emotional mind. It is often information held in the body that relates to adverse experiences in the form of repressed negative emotions and thoughts. When we gain a quiet mind, we also learn to process this information—the negative emotions and thinking that we have repressed—and experience it as simply sensation or energy. This will be emphasized in the exercises found in part 2, through which you will learn to observe information that is a source of chronic pain held inside of your body as energy and clear it.

Balance allows us to reduce allostatic load and handle stressors in a healthy way. When we are in balance, we can switch from the intellectual mind to the emotional mind to the overself. In balance we feel healthy because we are doing things to take care of ourselves every day. Taking care of ourselves includes practicing the exercises in this book, getting physical exercise, getting adequate rest, remaining intellectually curious, and reducing judgment, especially self-judgment.

Suffering

For our purposes, I define suffering as an experience of pain in which there is a sense of lost well-being. Suffering can have many causes. It can occur because of physical injury, emotional injury, chronic stress, increased allostatic load, and the inability to handle adversity.

As you have learned, when an experience occurs, we perceive and then interpret that experience. For example, as you read, you are perceiving the words on this page and you are interpreting their meaning. That interpretation has a story associated with it—a story of chronic pain and the hope of overcoming that chronic pain. That is your perception and interpretation in the moment. The interpretation allows you to understand an event, but the interpretation also forces you to make a judgment.

Most judgments are couched in a cause-and-effect paradigm. For example, when I exercise (the cause) I feel healthier (the effect). I then learn to associate feeling healthier with exercise (the judgment). As we discussed in chapter 10, when we perceive and interpret information, we frame that information, which allows us to give it a certain meaning. Part of the framing process involves our understanding of a cause-and-effect relationship. In the example above, cause and effect is pretty easy to determine. But now let's consider that an injury (cause) has produced pain (effect). Also consider that this pain now becomes the cause of impaired cognition and negative emotions. Over time that original pain becomes the *cause* of the ongoing pain and suffering, even though the original injury is no longer an issue. When cause-and-effect relationships are applied to chronic pain, the situation is indeed complex. In the case of chronic pain, pain can be both an effect and a cause. Let us look at this statement a little more closely.

I have made the argument that pain and suffering often occur as a result of the internalized somatic component of emotions that accompany adverse experiences. I have also previously stated that much of what we internalize can affect how we process present or future information. This occurs because the internalized somatic component of the emotion has a direct effect on our schemas (the rules that the mind uses to process information). The process works like this: We experience an adverse event, one that causes some level of pain. We internalize the somatic emotional components, storing the pain in our body. This alters our schemas so we make judgments that make it more likely that we will experience future events as negative and painful—a vicious cycle. In this way, the pain that started as an effect of some cause (an adverse event) now becomes the cause of future pain.

That is how chronic pain works. Our suffering is not only the effect of an adverse experience but is also the cause of future adverse experiences, or suffering. Try to remember the first time you experienced pain that was prolonged. The original pain may have been caused by an injury, but soon the pain itself caused a change in cognitions and emotional processing. If the pain became chronic, then you can imagine a vicious cycle of pain being both cause and effect, spiraling out of control.

The emotional component of suffering

Previously we discussed that every experience has an emotional component associated with it. I also stated that an emotion has a cognitive aspect and a somatic aspect. When we experience an emotion that is negative, the way we handle or process this emotion at the moment it is experienced has lasting impact—especially when the emotion is extremely negative. When one does not have the coping skills to properly process highly charged emotions, the somatic component of that emotion often remains in the body and gets trapped there. It is almost as though there is a somatic "tag" that gets stuck. This is where the problem of chronic pain often begins. The somatic part of the negatively charged emotion remains in the body. It alters our schemas and influences how future information is evaluated and framed on various levels:

- On the level of the *brain,* these alterations of our schemas, how we process information, can be seen by structural and functional changes in brain areas that process negative emotions.

- On the level of *stress,* this leads to a high allostatic load and continued present and chronic stress.

- On the level of the three *minds* (intellectual, emotional, and overself), it keeps us in the intellectual and emotional minds as we are constantly analyzing, are using residual emotional components in our interpretations, and do not have the ability to quiet our mind and go into the overself.

So when we are in chronic pain, negative emotional energy seems to be "stuck" in the body. It can alter our brain function, our capacity to handle stress (the allostatic load), and our intellectual and emotional processing. All of this interferes with our ability to reach the important overself mind, which is essential for releasing the burden. Working through the exercises in part 2 can change this by helping us practice putting attention on how the body feels and learning to experience sensations and energy that reside inside the body. But we have a few more things to learn before we begin practicing these techniques.

The concept of "trapped energy" and suffering

It may seem unusual to you that I am talking about something non-material, like emotions and thoughts, being "stuck," like the accumulation of energy in the body. In much of this book, I have talked about physical structures in the brain and body, and outcomes that we have been able to demonstrate through decades of research into phenomena such as the stress response in the brain and mind. But as for the idea of some sort of "energy" stuck in the body, well, there is no direct empirical evidence that this exists. However, the concept is deeply embedded in Chinese medicine, and even though we do not have proof in traditional Western science and medicine, we do have evidence that the methods based on this concept produce positive results. One of those methods, or practices, is the Chinese technique *Qigong* (pronounced "chee gung"), which I have practiced and used with my patients for many years. Qigong, an exercise technique that is over 5,000 years old, involves the use of Qi energy (the energy of life in Chinese medicine), movement, and breathing to achieve a quiet mind. When this energy is not strong and flowing well, one is open to chronic disease such as chronic pain. In my program, I do Qigong energy treatments on my patients and teach Qigong movement and mindfulness as well. As a practitioner, I have gained the ability to feel the negative energy in the form of trapped emotions from past adverse events in my patients and help them to clear it through my treatments. When I am able to do so, there is a significant change not only in the perceived pain but also in the balance of energy, and this has a dramatic impact on one's health.

The cognitive component of suffering

We have already learned that chronic pain influences the mind and brain, and it impacts the way we process present information. It does so by influencing our schemas (the rules by which we process this information in the mind). The cognitive component of chronic pain could be described as a thought process of suffering, and I believe that much of that suffering is brought on by our inability to process the somatic component of past and present adversity that gets stuck in our body. As a Qigong practitioner, I view this as energy that has been stuck and stagnated in the body. This concept may seem somewhat exotic to some readers, and while there is a growing body of research backing up the effectiveness of Qigong, to the uninitiated, it must be taken with some degree of faith, since it does not easily lend itself to traditional experimental techniques. If it is helpful, you may think of this as an adaptation of some accepted theoretical models of the brain-mind-body in Chinese medicine that have produced healing for centuries, but which Western science has not yet been able to document. I only ask that you keep an open mind.

Conclusion

As has been reviewed in this chapter, I believe that much of what causes people to suffer is the inability to properly process emotions. When this occurs, the energy, or Qi, that is associated with the somatic component of those emotions gets stuck inside of the body. This can influence the amount of stress we experience (our allostatic load), how we process information (our schemas), and what mind (intellectual, emotional, or overself) we stay in. Unless this energy is processed, we will never be able to gain access to the overself to achieve a quiet mind.

Most of the book thus far has been based on research and work with patients conducted by me, my colleagues, and others who are exploring alternatives to traditional chronic pain treatment. In this chapter, I have asked you to take something of a leap of faith to ready yourself to try the exercises in part 2, and to trust that techniques like Qigong have a long history of success in traditional Chinese medicine, even if we do not yet know how the process works.

The next chapter will cover the concept of coping—our ability to handle and address adversity.

• • •

14

Coping

Each day, we are confronted with stress, and in order to handle that stress, we must have the ability to cope. You are probably familiar with what it means to cope, but for this chapter I would like to give it a formal definition:

> *Coping* is the response that we have for dealing with adversity such as pain and stress.

> *Healthy coping* is the use of the sufficient energy required to deal with stress in the most efficient manner and with the least impact on our allostatic load ("stress basket").

Our ability to cope is a strong determinant of how well we will do in life. Our coping ability also determines how we will handle pain, especially if the pain is prolonged and becomes chronic. Personality plays an important role in how well we cope. Of course, like the word *cope,* we hear the term *personality* a lot, but it also needs a formal definition:

> *Personality* is the dynamic organization of psychological and physiological qualities that underlie an individual's patterns of thoughts, actions, and feelings.

More broadly, personality is what makes a person the individual that he or she is. Studies have shown that certain personality types are better at coping than others. For example, people with traits such as conscientiousness, extroversion, positive attitude (optimism), and openness to new challenges are more successful at coping with adversity. In contrast, people with traits such as anxiety, fear, moodiness, and worry are often less successful at coping.

Personality and coping are independent concepts, yet they are interactive and they can influence your response to adversity and your physical, mental, and spiritual health. The type of personality you have may determine how you cope with pain.

In this chapter, we will look at the relationship between coping and personality and will also explore how to identify your own coping style.

Coping with Adversity

Each time you attempt to accomplish a task, you use your ability to pay attention to the task and keep attention on that task. This ability is referred to as *cognitive control*. The executive areas of the brain (the prefrontal cortex) use cognitive control to allow our mind to make the best choice possible with the information and perceptions we have available at any given moment. Cognitive control mechanisms allow us to override impulses such as fear, anger, shame, avoidance, and craving.

For example, try to remember a time when you were embarrassed by something someone said. Your immediate reaction may have been to run away or to strike back verbally or physically. But instead, you considered things such as the situation, the other person's behavior, the context of the embarrassing comment, the potential consequences of your action, and your future goals. You made a better choice that fit the circumstances. This was you using cognitive control. Cognitive control involves the mental ability to consider the bigger picture, the broader concerns, and acting accordingly. Different people have different degrees of cognitive control, and the amount of control varies depending on other factors.

Impulsiveness can be described as the opposite of cognitive control, because to be impulsive means to act reflexively (without contemplation). For example, when one experiences emotional pain, the first impulse may be to seek the easiest way to avoid the pain at any cost and without consideration of consequences. In the example above, an impulsive person might have run off immediately (avoiding the emotional pain of embarrassment) or slapped the person (trying to avoid a future insult).

We have all had these experiences of what is called *avoidant behavior,* but by learning to use healthy coping skills that increase our cognitive control, we come to see that our old way of approaching the stressor (the pain) was, for the most part, responsible for the pain. We may also realize that much of the pain had been fueled by the anxiety our behavior provoked. Try looking back at some of the times you have used avoidant behavior and see if you can think of ways you could have used your cognitive control to create a better outcome.

Cognitive control mechanisms, for the most part, have *executive control privilege* in the brain. This means that they take precedence over and can inhibit any other thoughts or impulses. As noted above, cognitive control can gather sufficient mental resources to overcome most any adversity, but using cognitive control takes practice and, most important, *the motivation to practice.* The ability to override impulses and to act or think in an appropriate manner determines what we pay attention to and what we can accomplish. When we succeed at this, we are acting from our *I,* or *objective self,* and exercising our capacity for agency (taking action). When we gain the ability to control attention, we gain the ability to engage in situations that, at first, may be perceived as overly difficult, unachievable, and threatening. When we are able to take on situations that we once might have avoided, we can move forward in a goal-directed manner and avoid reflexive (or impulsive) behaviors. Using cognitive control helps us avoid poor decisions that can result from misperceptions of certain situations.

Goal-directed behaviors usually have *expectancies.* That is, we expect our action will result in an outcome that, to a great extent, can be predicted. However, not everything that is expected occurs, and when it does not, we often feel distress and pain. It is not always possible to predict when this will occur. So, for example, you may expect that your action of sending flowers to a friend will result in something in return for you, such as a thank you or increased feelings of goodwill between you and your friend. But let's say you send the flowers and get no thanks or no acknowledgment. That is an unexpected and unpredicted outcome of your goal-directed behavior. Your immediate reaction might be anger, feelings of rejection, or other emotional pain from lack of acknowledgment.

It is the ability to change or shift mentally (an ability called *cognitive flexibility*) that allows us to achieve a given goal despite the adversity that occurs when the expectancy is not predictable—that is, when what we expect does not occur. If, in the example above, you were a person who had inflexible thinking, you might stay in a state of anger and disappointment. But if you had the capacity to shift mentally and use cognitive flexibility, you might imagine other causes for your friend's lack of acknowledgment, from the flowers not arriving to your friend being ill, being out of town, or having another unknown problem. You might even realize that you could continue to care for your friend, even if your friend's actions were deliberately neglectful. *Cognitive control improves our ability to shift mentally when our expectations are not realized.* Without this ability, we become overburdened with failed attempts to achieve a goal. This can often lead to feelings of sadness, despair, isolation, inadequacy, and seeing ourselves as a failure. It can also cause us to avoid certain situations that may lead to negative feelings.

Cognitive control, cognitive flexibility, and chronic pain

Chronic pain reduces both cognitive control and cognitive flexibility, since chronic pain is often perceived as uncontrollable and untreatable. Recall from earlier chapters that people who have experienced both chronic pain and past adversity have a reduced capacity to exercise the kind of cognitive control I have just described. Constant stress has kept them in a fight-or-flight state for too long; their "stress basket" is overburdened or broken. This means they are more likely to be impulsive—to be unable to use the cognitive control just described. More real and perceived situations trigger stress, which means more pain, which they want to avoid, adding yet more stress due to the avoidance. Because the outcomes (expectancies) of new and novel experiences are less predictable, people with chronic pain are more likely to avoid such experiences. So, for example, when former college tennis player J. began experiencing severe back pain, the idea of trying to move in a new and novel way by sweeping her tennis racket very slowly in the same motion she had used to defeat challengers seemed like an activity to avoid. The outcome was unpredictable, and that unpredictability caused fear and stress. She was (at first) not open to the new and novel behavior.

Lack of openness to new behavior is a characteristic of people who have had chronic adversity, chronic stress, and chronic pain. This is understandable and has a certain sort of logic to it: new behaviors *are* likely to result in unfamiliar, unpredictable, and possibly unsuccessful outcomes. Yet the alternative is worse: repeating the same behaviors is only going to repeat the same or worse outcomes. Moreover, openness to new and novel experiences is essential to improving cognitive control and flexibility, thereby improving coping skills.

When people have become fearful of new experiences, they may nonetheless find the willingness to attempt them by becoming open to the idea that first attempts at novel experiences will simply not be successful and learn not to take this as a personal failure. We can also break up new activities into smaller, more achievable (less unpredictable) goals and plan sub-goals that can be flexible and changeable. *Sub-goals* are stepwise strategies that lead to the eventual attainment of a given goal. For example, J. could break her goal of returning to tennis play into many sub-goals. One might be to first rehearse her serve in her head, many times. That is a very predictable sub-goal. Presumably, it cannot hurt if it is only in her head. Or, her first goal could be to hold the racket and squeeze it gently. With flexible thought, any number of achievable sub-goals can be imagined that will help her begin to regain her lost confidence.

The ability to engage in sub-goals and disengage when the expectancy changes is an important aspect of our ability to cope and can lead to positive future experiences and help us avoid negative outcomes and emotions.

Coping and Stress

Successful coping becomes possible when we have the ability to handle stress. Stress can be viewed as the experience of adversity that often occurs during goal-directed behavior. We feel stress when faced with unanticipated outcomes, events, and consequences, which might ultimately lead to loss. (Of course, the unanticipated outcomes may lead toward gain, but we do not know—the outcomes are unpredictable.) To remain goal-directed, it is important to maintain the ability to overcome negative emotions such as frustration, anger, anxiety, and fear. We must be able to always stay focused on the big picture. Remember that the ability to inhibit negative emotions is a cognitive control mechanism. When we can inhibit those emotions, we are better able to make the best choice possible, to be thoughtful instead of impulsive, and to reduce the burden of stress.

There are different ways of responding to stress. These coping styles have varying impacts on stress, sometimes diminishing it but sometimes making it worse, depending on the response used. For people with chronic pain, choosing an appropriate coping response may help control pain and related anxiety.

Coping styles

When we encounter adversity, we have to make a decision about just *what* to pay attention to. For example, do we focus on the immediate problem at hand? The potential long-term consequences? Our feelings of fear and anxiety? Our attention can determine our coping styles. Coping styles include problem-focused coping, engagement coping, disengagement coping (also called avoidance), accommodation coping, meaning-focused coping, and proactive coping.

Problem-focused coping refers to the process of focusing on the problem that is causing the stress. When we use this coping style, we try to remove, evade, or diminish the impact of the stressor. If this is not possible, serious emotional distress may occur. Problem-focused coping is aimed at minimizing the stress and the accompanying feelings. It includes techniques like relaxation, self-soothing, seeking emotional support, or expressing negative emotions by means such as yelling and crying. When problem-focused coping is negative, it may involve a focus on negative thoughts, which can include rumination and catastrophic thinking. It may also involve avoidance, denial, and wishful thinking.

The nature of problem-focused coping often depends on the goal that the coping is intended to achieve. For example, if our goal is to gain emotional support, then we express the emotions associated with the stressor. This can serve to diminish negative stress and make it possible to consider the problem from a more calm and logical perspective, often leading to better problem-focused coping.

Engagement coping refers to using a process that actively engages the stressor and relies on our ability to deal with stress and related negative emotions. Engagement coping includes strategies such as problem solving and reframing (discussed in chapter 10). Engagement coping may involve seeking emotional support, emotional regulation, acceptance, and reassessing the situation.

Disengagement coping often involves avoidance, in which we seek to avoid the pain and the negative emotions associated with the stressor. We attempt to escape the perceived threat and related emotion. This method of coping may include responses such as denial, wishful thinking, avoiding the feelings brought on by stress and pain, or pretending the stressor does not exist or will just go away, thereby distancing ourselves from the stressful situation. Unfortunately, disengagement only leads to internalization and more pain (the stressor never goes away). It is generally ineffective in reducing stress, and it does nothing about the continued existence of the stressor, how it is perceived, and the eventual outcome. For example, if a person is experiencing a stressor and responds by getting stoned or drunk, then the stressor is still there after the individual sobers up. Often the longer we avoid dealing with the problem, the more challenging it becomes and the fewer options remain available to deal with it when we finally attempt to do so.

Paradoxically, avoidance often can lead to an *increase* in intrusive thoughts about the stress or an increase in negative mood, anxiety, and emotions. Disengagement can also lead to increased pain; increased avoidant behavior, such as drug misuse, shopping, or gambling; and diminished quality of social, physical, and mental health. These can have negative health and financial consequences. Disengagement coping can cause us to give up goals and settle for much less in an attempt to avoid failure and distress. It can also cause us to further avoid and pull back from life experiences. All of these consequences add up to an increase in negative feelings, which can lead to more pain.

Accommodation coping refers to attempts to control and adjust to stress. Accommodation involves the ability to adjust inner feelings and strategies in order to handle the stressors. This style may involve self-constraint and modulation of, or adjusting, our feelings. Self-constraint involves monitoring our thoughts, actions, and behaviors through the use of cognitive control. In order to do this, we must have the ability to monitor our internal thoughts before they become reflexive (automatic reactions). This takes practice and it can be a healthy behavior, as in not giving in to rage when trying to resolve conflict with someone, or a defensive survival behavior, as when adjusting and suppressing feelings to avoid abuse. Modulation of feelings involves monitoring our internal feelings and emotions through cognitive control. This also takes practice, as we need to develop the ability to monitor internal sensations. Reframing the situation and adjusting goals are two other forms of accommodation that are most useful.

Meaning-focused coping attempts to extract positive meaning from the stressful situation. One aspect of meaning-focused coping is the ability to use attention in a focused manner. When a person is able to put attention on the relevant aspects of the stressor and evaluate the positive aspects of having experienced that stressor, he or she can derive positive meaning from the experience. For example, some people routinely explore how a particular experience—even a negative one—has helped them grow and learn. This activity helps them bring meaning to a stressful or painful event. This practice can be enhanced by using positive feedback and positive emotions and feelings to clarify the interpretation or meaning derived from the stressor.

Proactive coping refers to preparing for a likely stressor. This approach helps us defuse threatening or harmful situations before they occur. It is generally problem-focused and involves accumulating useful resources in order to control the emotions and cognition associated with the situations preceding the stressful event. Proactive coping allows us to anticipate future outcomes and approach them in such a way so that they will not be overwhelming and cause undue stress. This method of coping also includes strategies to keep threats from escalating, so that if a threat is perceived we are able to engage in cognitive control and avoid the perception of an expanding threat.

For example, even when we have brought chronic pain under control, we must prepare to experience pain in the future. When any new pain comes, all the fears and feelings associated with the chronic pain come rushing back. Proactive coping in this instance means preparing to use cognitive control and reframing to adjust negative thoughts and emotions previously linked with chronic pain. With proactive coping, we have a plan ready for future pain, and that plan enables us to handle and diminish the pain—to cope with the pain in a healthy way rather than responding with fear, avoidance, and more pain.

Now take some time to determine which of the coping strategies you engage in:

- problem-focused coping
- engagement coping
- disengagement coping (also called avoidance)
- accommodation coping
- meaning-focused coping
- proactive coping

Think of times you may have used each of these coping strategies. Then, ask yourself, Was this coping strategy an automatic response to the event or person triggering the stress, or was it chosen by me? That is, do you control your choice of coping strategy or does the stressor control it?

Most of us have collected many of these coping strategies in our cognitive toolkit. If certain coping strategies become habitual, then often they are hard to recognize. That is why it is important to expose yourself to novel situations and then try to identify how you cope with those situations.

Personality Traits and Coping

As you can see, there are a variety of ways to cope with adversity and stress, and some of these are more effective than others. But why do some people cope differently than others? We all know people who seem to view even major setbacks as opportunities rather than losses. And we all know people for whom a paper cut is a day-wrecker. Clearly, these two groups of people have very different ways of seeing and interpreting events in their worlds. Though not completely anchored in personality, the ways we perceive and frame events are related to personality traits. Certain personality traits are connected with successful coping, while others are linked with unsuccessful coping. We will review these personality traits first and then examine their influence on coping.

Personality traits

Just as an artist can mix a few colors into an endless variety of shades and hues, humans seem to mix a few personality traits into a variety of behaviors and ways of experiencing and interpreting the world. Below are some traits that occur in human personality that you will no doubt recognize in yourself and others. These traits include extroversion (or "outgoingness"), neuroticism (a tendency to experience negative emotions), agreeableness (a tendency to be compassionate and friendly), conscientiousness (being organized and dependable), optimism (looking on the bright side), and openness to new experience (or curiosity).

Extroversion, also thought of as "being outgoing," is associated with assertiveness and the positive use of energy. It may be perceived as dominance, confidence, agency, and sociability. The general approach we use to carry out a plan goes far in determining whether or not we are extroverts. For instance, extroverts seldom avoid situations when attempting to accomplish a given plan. These characteristics usually help a person cope well with adverse events.

Neuroticism is characterized by anxiety, fear, moodiness, worry, envy, frustration, jealousy, depression, and isolation. Neurotic people become upset and distressed quite easily. They often experience anxiety from misperceiving a situation as a threat (for example, viewing a stranger's glance as an imminent attack). In this way, neuroticism has been linked to avoidance and the tendency to disengage when a situation becomes difficult. In certain cases, neuroticism is also associated with low self-esteem and very high, difficult expectations for oneself. These expectations are often quite different from the expectations the individuals place on others. A neurotic person does not easily cope with stress.

Agreeableness is the ability to be friendly, helpful, and understanding and to try to please others while inhibiting negative feelings and emotions. People who are agreeable are generally willing to consider and understand the viewpoints of others. People who are agreeable get less angry over the actions of others and less angry at those who do not agree with them. They typically can tolerate behaviors that they perceive to be different from theirs, not well thought out, or senseless. Agreeableness can have a negative side, however, such as when people just go along with others and do not express their own preferences or repress their real feelings. At the opposite end of agreeableness are oppositional and antagonistic qualities and the inability to deal with social conflict.

Conscientiousness is the ability to constrain impulses and negative behaviors while proceeding in a responsible, reflective, and reliable manner. Agreeableness and conscientiousness have much in common. Both suggest that one has a wide and open perspective. When people remain open to experience, they are able to be good students and remain inquisitive and continue to learn while not shutting out experiences that they may perceive as unpleasant or threatening. These qualities lead to improvement of thought and intellect. They also relate to curiosity, flexibility, imagination, and the willingness to immerse oneself in experiences that are personal and social. Conscientiousness is associated with good coping skills.

Optimism (keeping a positive outlook) involves confidence and the ability to see the good in things and people. It allows one to look beyond a specific negative experience while remembering that positive aspects will come with future experiences. Optimism can be contrasted with pessimism, the belief that things are most likely to turn out poorly. Optimism is an important quality that leads to successful coping and can dramatically decrease one's experience of pain.

Openness to experience and change is a general sense of curiosity about the world. It includes being open to emotional experience, sensitive to beauty, and willing to try new things. People who are not open to experience tend to prefer familiar situations over new ones, and may resist change.

How personality traits influence coping

Our personality traits influence how frequently we expose ourselves to stressful experiences, the type of stressful experiences we are willing to encounter, and how we perceive those experiences. No one person has all one trait and none of another. We all have a mix of traits, and the combinations can affect how we cope with stress.

Extroversion has been associated with sensitivity to reward, positive emotions, sociability, and assertiveness. These traits help people engage persistently in problem solving. It can also cause stress if extroverts are too dependent on external rewards for their sense of worth. Extroverts have the ability to change the way they process information so that it is more adaptive to stressors. Thus, they can change cognitive schemas. This ability to restructure cognitive schemas and change the way they view others helps extroverts develop strong social networks and social support, which also help with coping.

Neuroticism, the tendency toward negative emotions, predicts exposure to personal stress and the tendency to appraise events as highly threatening. This will be accompanied by coping resources that are generally poor or not available. People who are high in neuroticism and low in conscientiousness (the ability to plan and be dependable) are also more likely to experience larger loads of stress and to perceive more situations as threatening. Neuroticism is associated with fear, sadness, distress, and high states of physiological arousal. People who tend toward neuroticism often focus on emotional coping and disengagement coping. Disengagement may be perceived as short-term relief from the stress. The presence of intense emotional arousal can interfere with the use of engagement strategies that require careful planning. Negative emotions can make positive thinking and cognitive restructuring difficult.

Agreeableness, the tendency to be compassionate and friendly, is associated with low interpersonal conflict and therefore less social stress, except when being agreeable is a ploy to avoid conflict; in that case it can cause more stress. However, agreeableness generally requires having high levels of trust and concern for others. It often predicts one's level of social support. More social support may make more coping resources available when faced with adversity.

Conscientiousness tends to cause people to experience more stress. This probably occurs because many people who are conscientious have higher expectations of themselves and put themselves in more stressful situations. However, they also plan for predictable exposure to stressful situations and avoid impulsive actions. This can lead to fewer problems with relationships, finances, and health. The ability to regulate emotion is strongly associated with conscientiousness. Therefore, people with this trait are more likely to succeed at reframing and also find it easier to disengage from or inhibit negative thoughts.

Optimism involves the expectation that good outcomes will come from good efforts. Optimism relates positively to coping styles that include problem solving and reframing. Of all of the personality traits, optimism has consistently been shown to be the best and most adaptive. In contrast, people who are pessimistic (expect poor outcomes) are more likely to use disengagement or avoidance as a coping strategy.

Openness, or being open to new experiences, often involves being imaginative, creative, curious, flexible, and highly aware of one's inner feelings toward new activities and ideas. An openness to explore and experience new coping strategies can have a positive effect on how we deal with stressors. When people are open to changing their coping strategy, they become willing to find the best way to deal with a given stressor.

Of course, these traits can work together to influence whether we see events as opportunities or threats; they can shape the way we cope with adversity, whether we cope by disengaging and avoidance or by engaging and problem solving; and they can affect how we expect our efforts to turn out. Extroversion, conscientiousness, and openness are all associated with the ability to perceive events as a challenge rather than a threat. These traits are also associated with the ability to appraise a given situation positively and to use positive coping resources.

People who respond to a stressor by active engagement use approaches that involve reframing their thoughts, perceptions, and strategies. This is why traits such as optimism, openness, agreeableness, conscientiousness, and extroversion are helpful. An optimistic person predicts a positive outcome for one's actions, and a conscientious person plans and regulates emotions. An agreeable person will have more social supports to cope with any emotional stress and will be able to see the stressful event with more compassion for others as well. These traits make it easier to reframe thoughts and perceptions while regulating emotions and planning for the next goals.

In contrast, neuroticism influences people to cope with stress by disengaging rather than through reframing and emotional regulation. Disengagement coping is associated with strategies of denial, substance use, and other avoidance tactics such as wishful thinking and withdrawal. Disengagement coping is also connected with a greater perception of pain and an inability to handle pain.

So, as you can see, different traits combine in various ways to influence our coping style in fascinating ways. But we have some control over our responses.

Conclusion

A relationship has been established between mental health, physical health, personality traits, and coping strategies. People whose traits tend more strongly toward extroversion, conscientiousness, agreeableness, openness, and optimism are more likely to cope well with stress. In contrast, people who tend toward neuroticism, anxiety, and depression are more likely to rely on maladaptive coping strategies. These traits have also been associated with chronic pain and substance misuse.

The ability to draw on adaptive coping strategies during times of adversity or stress will determine future success at releasing the burden of chronic pain. It is important that you begin to analyze what coping strategies you use to handle stressors and how these strategies influence your internal states. If you are able to engage in cognitive control mechanisms that lead to successful coping strategies, your ability to handle pain will be significantly enhanced.

You have learned a lot in this chapter about how people cope with stress and how personality interacts with coping style. It is not as though you have to change your personality, though. We all possess some level of each of these traits. We can learn to nudge ourselves closer to one trait or another and, in so doing, begin to use more adaptive coping styles. This is one reason that I suggested back in chapter 9 that you begin practicing a simple breathing exercise. As I said, this exercise will help you experience your "overself" mind. This, along with other mindfulness exercises in part 2, will help you learn to observe your current coping strategies and emotional reactions so you can begin to navigate them in more adaptive directions.

Identifying your personality traits and honestly appraising your coping style is an important step toward learning to deal with chronic pain. In the next chapter, you will take another step in that direction as we complete our preparations for the exercises. We noted that the best coping strategy for people with chronic pain is optimism expressed in the idea that you can overcome pain. The exercises in part 2 are designed to help you gain confidence and the optimism that you can become pain free.

• • •

15

Feeling

A book on chronic pain would be incomplete without a discussion of the ability to feel. The word *feeling* means different things depending on the specific context, so let's begin with a definition.

> In this book, **feeling** means perceiving sensations or energy inside of your body.

This definition is important because, as we discussed throughout the book, adversity has a tremendous impact on the amount of pain you feel, how that pain influences you, and the development of chronic physical pain. Yet, most of the time, when you ask people with chronic pain how they feel, they have a difficult time responding beyond saying, "I hurt." All they can tell you about is the sensation of pain, since they do not feel anything else. Many of them are out of touch with most other feelings, and yet, the body is home to a wide array of feelings.

As you will soon begin the exercises, it is important to understand that there is an abundance of information residing within your body, but that information has no intellectual interpretation; it is simply an experience. By this I mean it is not a function of the intellectual mind. Instead, it is a function of the overself.

I hope that you have been practicing the breathing exercise that I described in chapter 9 and that this exercise has allowed you to begin to know what it is to escape from the intellectual mind and place your attention on sensations and energy inside your body. Through working the additional mindfulness exercise in part 2, you will learn to quiet the mind and become more adept at focusing your attention on what you feel inside your body. This is a very important endeavor but, after years of being at the mercy of the demands of your intellectual mind and emotional mind on a daily basis, it takes time to be able to experience a quiet mind. It is not that being in the emotional and intellectual minds is a bad thing. As we learned earlier, they both serve their purpose and are a part of who you are. The problem develops when this is the only way you know your body and the world, especially when your thoughts and feelings have been hijacked by the adversity in your life. Be patient with yourself and trust the innate wisdom of your brain-mind-body to be aware and heal itself.

So let's go ahead and describe exactly what it means to "feel things" inside your body. From there, we will look at what prevents us from feeling.

Exteroception Versus Interoception

Let's recap some key ideas from earlier chapters. Our brain and mind are equipped with the ability to take in information from the environment. This ability is called perception, and our brain has specific areas that allow us to perceive the world. It is such an important function that the brain has an entire lobe dedicated to vision, and important parts of different lobes are dedicated to hearing, taste, smell, and touch.

There are at least two environments from which we can perceive—the external world (sensations around us) and the internal world (sensations inside us).

The process of perceiving sensations from the external world is called *exteroception.* We are blessed with the abilities to see, to hear, to touch and feel, to taste, and to smell. Thus, we have access to a wealth of information from which we can extract data to be processed in our mind and brain. If you consider it, there is so much information in our external environment that the brain and mind must be able to focus our attention on those aspects that are judged to be most important. If we lacked this ability, our mind would experience chaos—an overload of information. Thus, our brain and mind have the ability to select which aspects of the external environment to attend to and, in this way, are able to meet our needs and goals at any given time.

We also have the ability to place our attention on the environment that exists inside of our body—the internal environment. This process is referred to as *interoception.* There is a wealth of information inside our body at all times, but most of us seldom pay attention to it. This can be a problem, especially when we have chronic pain, because it is as we learn to attend to this internal environment and the information available to us that healing can occur. The proof that true healing is possible will be evident in the transformation that occurs when you begin to do the exercises and make them part of your life. Some people are not able to attend to their internal environment because they never learned it was important (especially in our externally focused material culture) or were afraid of what they would find there; others have had times when they were in touch with themselves on that level, but they have been distracted by their suffering or their fascination with the external world and have lost that ability. This is especially true for people with chronic pain. Now, let's look at why people are not able to perceive the environment that exists inside of the body.

Why Can't I Feel?

I often ask patients why they can't feel—why they are poor at feeling sensations inside of their body. Interestingly, most have never considered this question before, nor have they ever considered how important it is to be able to focus their attention on how it feels inside their body. Although we are born with this natural ability, we probably do not pay attention to it for very long after we "grow up." Instead we become externally focused and lose the ability to attend to our inner sensations very well.

Another reason we may lose touch with this natural ability is that our internal perceptions may seem too difficult for us to cope with. This may be especially true for people who have been overwhelmed by adversity. A typical coping mechanism, as noted in chapter 14, is avoidance. We tend to choose avoidance when we have a very painful experience that carries with it the pain of a negative emotion. The somatic component attached to that emotion may be too much for us, and so we decide to ignore the feelings inside our body. We talked about how this approach causes a tremendous amount of suffering. Yet the continued conscious or unconscious attempt to avoid perceiving sensations and energy inside of the body is both the cause and the effect of continued chronic pain.

Consistently, when I go around the room during pain groups and ask people how much attention they put on the messages that exist inside of their body, the response is basically none—there is only pain and they prefer not to be conscious of it. They pay no attention at all to other messages and so all that they perceive is the sensation of pain, and they ignore or deny the wealth of other information inside of them.

I suspect that one part of this problem is that at a very early age, we are put into a system of education that stresses the development of the intellectual mind. To be sure, we must attend to our own and our children's intellectual development, and maintaining intellectual curiosity throughout life is a key to positive neuroplasticity. However, if we ignore the signals inside of our body, it will be just a matter of time until our allostatic load becomes overwhelming and chronic stress becomes unavoidable. What's more, ignoring the internal environment affects our schemas—how our mind programs the information it receives. This occurs because internalized emotions cause stress and influence how we process information so that the brain is, for the most part, reflexive rather than thoughtful and reflective.

As we begin the exercises in part 2, it is important to understand that, by learning to read these messages, you can begin to return your body to its capacity to release the stress and burdens you carry and to find a state of balance.

Why Don't I *Want* to Feel?

Somewhere along the way in life, we may have decided not to put our attention on the messages that are inside of us; essentially, we are saying that we do not want to feel.

After observing chronic pain patients for over ten years, I have concluded that many of them have come to believe that attending to inner feelings will be painful. They are stuck in an autobiographical narrative that frames these inner feelings as painful, and that is where the pain exists: *it is in the narrative.* Remember, the autobiographical narrative is the home of interpretation and judgment, and for people with chronic pain, those interpretations and judgments are, for the most part, negative.

It is not inherently painful to put attention on the information that exists inside of the body. That information consists only of sensations and energy. Yet we often choose to stay in the autobiographical narrative where all the pain is. For people with chronic pain, this is a story that has no other message except pain. There is no judgment in the energy of sensations that exist inside the body, but there is a wealth of judgment in the autobiographical narrative. Shifting attention to those sensations and energy is the focus of the exercises that you are about to begin.

Conclusion

We are now concluding the informational and theoretical portion of this book. Thank you for hanging in there with me! We have covered a lot of new and often complex terms and ideas, but what it all boils down to is one simple lesson: you have the ability within you to return to a life without chronic pain.

Let's review how we got here. You will recall that when pain becomes chronic, there is usually no direct relationship between tissue damage and pain. The disease of chronic pain is a disease of the brain and mind, and we reviewed specific aspects of the brain and mind that are affected by chronic pain. There are changes in the structure and function of the brain as well as changes in the schemas the mind uses to process information.

Chronic stress and present stress caused by adversity throughout life profoundly affect the development of chronic pain. Stress also has a significant effect on our autobiographical narrative, making it negative with little optimism. We should have the ability to choose which mind we want to be in, but chronic pain tends to keep us in the intellectual or emotional mind. It takes us away from the overself, that part of our mind that is able to objectively and calmly observe our sensations, thoughts, and emotions. Chronic pain limits the important component of cognitive control, and this limits our flexibility.

Most important, the brain-mind-body has the ability to heal if we are in balance. But if we want this to occur, we must practice gaining balance.

It may seem as though you have had to go back to school just to get ready to do a few exercises. Let me assure you, the reason for presenting all this information has not been for you to learn a lot of new ideas for their own sake! All of the things you have been learning have been preparing your brain and mind to benefit from the exercises in the second part of this book. I have learned from my patients that understanding just what goes on in the brain, mind, and body makes the exercises easier to practice.

As we continue on, one of the main focuses of the exercises will be to attain a quiet mind. Much of the reason we have great difficulty achieving a quiet mind is that we have internalized painful emotions; they are stuck inside us. Treating this condition is the primary goal of traditional Chinese medicine, and it is my goal as a Qigong practitioner. It is not your fault that you are in chronic pain, that you are out of touch with some painful feelings and experiences, that you live mostly in your intellectual and emotional minds, that you have an autobiographical narrative that tends to give a negative cast to all information. This is all a function of things that have happened to you, ways you have been taught (or not been taught) to cope, and lots of other factors. Even thinking that "It's all my fault" is a part of that pattern, and it is time to let go of this. The exercises will help.

The only requirement to be successful with these exercises is that you are dedicated to doing them consistently and you choose to take time for them every day. They have the ability to change your life. I have seen this happen for many people, and I have seen it happen in myself.

Let's move on and conquer chronic pain and suffering!

• • •

Part II: How We Heal

EXERCISES

Introduction to the Exercises

The exercises that follow are specifically designed to help you conquer chronic pain. Most are based on the philosophy of Qigong (pronounced "chee gung"), a Chinese discipline that integrates physical postures, breathing, mental focus, and a focus on energy. The others are "thinking" exercises that will prepare you to begin the more experiential exercises.

Before we get into the exercises themselves, let's explore some of the principles upon which these exercises are based.

The first principle is that the brain, mind, and body have the ability to heal.

The second principle is that you can use your ability to heal by observing energy or Qi (pronounced "chee"). *Qi* means "life energy."

The third principle is that healing requires you to quiet your mind by using breath and movement. Movement can be either the movement of your body or the movement of energy in your body. Since it is not practical to teach you how to move in a book, we will focus on the movement of energy.

The fourth principle is that one must learn to do passive observation. This means to simply observe by letting information come to you through direct experience. To do this, it is necessary to quiet your mind and be willing to heal. When your mind is quiet, you will allow the body's natural mechanism to heal itself. When you have achieved a quiet mind, you can allow information to come to you instead of seeking it in the intellectual mind.

The fifth principle is that you must allow yourself to heal. This is done by stopping active control, quieting the mind, and allowing yourself to use your natural mechanisms to heal.

The sixth principle is that you must learn to use intention. *Intention* is simply having the will or the aim for something to happen. This is not referring to an intentional act in which you actively engage in a process.

It is subtle in that all you have to do is have an intention to heal, quiet the mind, and allow the healing process to occur. Remember, the brain-mind-body wants to heal, and the intention to heal is the most important thing any of us can bring with us as we enter this path.

If you can quiet your mind, quiet the stress response, and observe energy, your pain will no longer be the primary focus of your attention. The exercises are designed to help you achieve a balanced mind, brain, body, and spirit. Do not worry if some of this does not make sense right now. These principles will become clearer as you actually do the exercises.

In order for the exercises to be effective, you must make the decision to practice them regularly. You must also make the decision that you are going to allow your body to heal. This means giving up judgment and control and just allowing your body to use its inherent mechanisms to heal. The body has an intelligence, much like the mind has an intelligence, but in order for the body to use its intelligence to heal, you must quiet your mind. When your mind is active in judgment and evaluation, it gets in the way and keeps you in the emotional or intellectual mind. This limits your ability to heal.

I have noted which exercises are most effective when practiced every day and which can be done on an as-needed basis. You can use exercise 6, Breath, as the basis for the other daily exercises. Simply add the other exercises as you become more acquainted with them and comfortable performing them.

Exercises 1 through 4 are preparatory exercises that will be helpful in the beginning as you are gaining insight about what may be keeping you in pain and how you can begin to clear the burden and quiet your mind. Let us begin.

• • •

EXERCISE 1:
PAIN CONFRONTED

We begin our exercises by learning to confront pain. You may have allowed pain to take control of your life. That is what pain does. It is not your fault, but eventually you grow tired of it. You may have been told by a professional that pain is permanent and cannot be conquered. However, in this book, you have learned that pain is a disease of the brain, body, and mind. Moreover, the brain, body, and mind can change and, in fact, have a great potential for change. We can help strengthen the body, but ultimately the brain and mind are what we must change. You must become an active participant in this process. This exercise will help you get started.

Pain Confronted Exercise

I want you to imagine that the poem below is chronic pain talking directly to you. I want you to feel the emotions that it causes within you when you read it. In order to do this, you must look at pain as an entity that can be confronted and one that can be overcome. Pain should be viewed as an enemy. Here is the poem, which my wife and I wrote about ten years ago.

CHRONIC PAIN

I am your pain.
You have let me in, and
I am here to stay.
I will consume you
and your energy
and your thoughts.
I will control your life;
I will never leave;
I will not allow you to be yourself;
I will control your emotions;
I will steal your sleep;

I will take you from your family;

I will steal you from your friends.

At times you may feel like I have left,

but I will always return.

I will show you no respect,

But you must respect me.

I will make you anxious.

I will make you uncertain.

When you are down, I will intensify.

I will make you feel alone;

I will destroy your sense of worth;

Your happiness is controlled by me;

There is no escape.

No one understands what I have done to you.

I can make you feel hopeless.

Confront me before it is too late.

Now it is time for you to respond. Go to a safe place away from other people where you can be alone. Close your eyes and allow yourself to access the emotions that this poem made you feel. Now tell pain exactly what you feel, as though it is standing or sitting directly in front of you. You are allowed to yell, scream, or pound a pillow, to become as emotional as needed. Do not hold back any of the sadness and anger, and do not hold back any other emotions that you experience. If it will help, ask someone you know and trust, such as a spouse/partner, relative, good friend, or counselor, to sit in front of you and imagine that this person is pain. Be sure that this is someone with whom you are completely comfortable. If you are concerned about the person's reactions to the intensity of your emotions—or if you think that you may need professional help in dealing with these feelings—you can do this exercise with a competent therapist. You can say anything you want to your pain. We have spoken a lot in the book about not judging and giving up control, but for this exercise you should judge pain and express your emotions.

How often to practice: Do this exercise as often as necessary until you feel that you can honestly confront pain, are no longer afraid of it, and feel that it is no longer going to control you. You can also find an outlet for these feelings through creative expression, such as music, drawing, or physical exertion to the degree that you are able to move. You are going to fight back with a plan that is going to defeat pain.

·

This exercise helps you switch your self-perception from someone who passively receives pain to someone who is proactive and ready to fight pain.

• • •

EXERCISE 2:
INTRODUCTION TO SCHEMAS

As you may recall, schemas are the rules that the mind uses to process information. Schemas can be dramatically altered by adverse events, past pain, and current pain. It is important that you begin trying to identify how your schemas may have been altered because if they are not working optimally, they compound suffering. This happens because your autobiographical narrative becomes increasingly negative and associated with suffering and pain.

Schema Exercise

Pages 191 and 192 contain two lists of words. The first group are skewed positively and the rest are skewed negatively. Once a day, review the words and rate how often you have thoughts and feelings during the day that are associated with those words. The ratings we will use are: often, sometimes, and never.

This exercise will help you understand how your mind processes information and how that processing may be contributing to pain. If much of your day is associated with the negatively skewed words, it is time to become aware of that and actively use your ability to change your thoughts and overcome these types of schemas.

You should begin to change the thoughts associated with words that have a negative connotation. To do this, first notice the negative thoughts and then place your attention on a positive thought. This is how you practice using *cognitive control:* the ability to place your attention on what you want. Use cognitive control to shift your thinking toward more positive and optimistic aspects of your life. We will practice this more in the next exercise. For now, just begin to recognize how often during the day your thoughts are positive or negative by using the list below. At the end of each day, put a tally mark in the correct box for each word. In the example, the person was often mindful one day during the week and not mindful at all the remaining six days.

Schema Exercise

	often	sometimes	never
Mindful *(example)*	I		̶I̶H̶I̶ I
Mindful			
Introspective			
Resilient			
Rested			
Sense of purpose			
Positive attitude			
Coping effectively with stress			
Forgiving of self			
Desire to change			
Focused on present			
Improved energy			
Optimistic			
Interoception (aware of your interior world)			
Empathetic			
Quiet mind			
Confident			
Sense of peace/connected			

Schema Exercise *continued*

	often	sometimes	never
Catastrophizing (predicting the worst)			
Fear of pain			
Hopeless			
Intellectualizing			
Stressed			
Reflexive thoughts			
Anxious			
Tired			
Dread the future			
Angry			
Harsh self-judgment			
Coping poorly with stress			
Sad			
Negative internal dialogue			
Negative thoughts of self			
Ruminating			
Self-doubt			
Without purpose			

How often to practice: Practice this exercise every day for the first month that you are doing these exercises. By then, you should be able to easily identify your thoughts that have a negative connotation.

•

This exercise is designed to help you see how much time you are spending with negative thought processes. The emotions associated with those negative thoughts are likely contributing to your suffering.

• • •

EXERCISE 3:
OVERCOMING NEGATIVE SCHEMAS

When negative schemas are influencing your thoughts, it is helpful to be in touch with the sensations that occur inside your body. In most cases, the sensations you feel will be those that are uncomfortable. You will also begin to realize that when you are repeating the same thoughts (i.e., ruminating) associated with negative schemas, those thoughts often carry a negative connotation (i.e., catastrophizing).

Changing Schemas Exercise

In this exercise, you will try to change the schemas that shape your thoughts and your narrative. Consider how much time you are spending with thoughts associated with the positive and negative words in exercise 2, Introduction to Schemas. For those words that have a negative connotation (the second group of words in *italics*), try to understand the schemas that generate your associated thought.

The next time you notice that your current thoughts are associated with a schema that is skewed negatively, actively stop yourself and realize that you are using a negative schema. For example, if you are facing a new experience—perhaps a new boss is joining the workforce—and you keep repeating the thoughts about all that could go wrong, you are ruminating. Recognize that you are ruminating. If you are faced with a new task and tell yourself you will likely fail, you are experiencing self-doubt, a negative internal narrative, negative thoughts of self, and harsh self-judgment. Recognize that you are doing this.

How often to practice: Practice this exercise until you understand it and then use it every time you become aware of yourself using a negative schema; it will take a few weeks before you become good at recognizing your negative schemas. As you do this, you will change your life by releasing much of the burden associated with rumination, catastrophic thinking, and any other negative schemas you have been using.

•

In this exercise, you are using cognitive control to overcome negative schemas that are contributing to pain. Use your ability to be in control of your attention to overcome negative schemas and allow yourself to reframe how you view and interpret the world.

• • •

EXERCISE 4:
WHO IS IN CONTROL?

Often, people with chronic pain try to control as much of their environment as they can. This behavior usually arises from the false belief that when we control more, we are protecting ourselves more. In reality, our attempts at control usually only worsen the situation.

Stop Control and Judgment Exercise

This exercise will teach you to be in the moment, an aspect of mindfulness.

Close your eyes and simply try to imagine what it is like to give up control, if only for one second. In order to do so, you will need to give up judgment and evaluation. Just allow yourself, even if it is for but a second, to stop judging and trying to control. See how that feels. You may feel a great sense of freedom right away or it may take a few attempts.

How often to practice: Practice this exercise until you begin to feel a sense of freedom.

• • •

EXERCISE 5:
THE MIND AND MINDFULNESS

I previously talked about how the thoughts and emotions generated by our personal narrative interfere with our ability to experience our actual sensations when the mind is quiet. We also discussed the overself and what it feels like to have a quiet mind. As you continue with these exercises, you will learn how to achieve a quiet mind by using the breath and viewing the energy inside your body.

Mind Exercise

Close your eyes and observe your thoughts. Simply allow the thoughts to pass into and through your mind and observe them. Try to look at your thoughts as though you are viewing a movie. Just get a sense of what it feels like to observe thoughts instead of being immersed in them.

How often to practice: Practice this exercise daily until you get a good sense of what it feels like to just view your thoughts.

•

This exercise is essential, as it will help you develop a sense of what it is like to just observe and not identify. Your mind likely often runs on its own and gives you the feeling that you are not in control.

Mindfulness is a very important aspect of conquering chronic pain. This involves the ability to put your attention on the present moment *without judgment* or attachment. Without judgment means without attaching a negative or positive label to the narrative—just neutral observation. Without attachment means without allowing it to become loaded with skewed emotions, especially negative ones that are painful. In other words, mindfulness is the ability to observe from the third-person perspective. This is close to the pure experiencing perspective of the overself.

Mindfulness Exercise

Now, begin to observe your thoughts for content and meaning, and see how they affect the way you feel. Try for one second to close your eyes and view yourself without any judgment or attachment. Observe how that feels. Some people get the feeling that they are suddenly falling—almost as though they have tumbled off a cliff and are falling freely through the air. If you cannot do this exercise without feeling too uncomfortable to continue, you might enlist the help of a meditation group or teacher or a counselor who is familiar with meditation practices to guide you through it until you can view your thoughts. It is best to enlist one who is familiar with Qigong.

How often to practice: Practice viewing your thoughts without judgment as often as you can throughout the day until it feels comfortable. This will bring you closer to achieving a mindful state. Remember to be conscious of any self-judgment when doing this exercise. We can even find ourselves judging our judgment, and adding extra layers of unnecessary stress. When this happens, just step back and, with detachment, simply observe these thoughts and any emotions they cause.

•

Becoming mindful and stopping judgment are important to releasing the burden of chronic pain. From this perspective, you will not judge your experience, which means you will not be attaching negative schemas or negative narratives, or otherwise reinforcing the cycle of pain. You will therefore have nothing to avoid, and you can regain contact with past experiences that became stored in your body.

This practice allows you to ground yourself and be present throughout the day and provides a foundation for the exercises that follow.

• • •

EXERCISE 6:
BREATHING

Now is an appropriate time to formally begin using the breathing exercise that was introduced in part 1, chapter 9. Hopefully, you have been doing this exercise regularly, as was recommended, and are ready to add it to the more formal exercise program that you have now begun. Breathing is an important aspect of the energy work that you will begin with exercise 11 because it is a good entry point to help you quiet the mind and begin to view energy. You can practice your other daily exercises when you perform the breathing exercise, adding the other exercises as they are introduced. When you achieve a quiet mind, you are able to place attention on the sensations that are inside your body and to realize that what you are viewing is energy.

Breathing Exercise 1
(This is the same exercise that you learned in chapter 9.)

Close your eyes, sit up straight in a chair with your feet on the floor, and place your hands in a comfortable position. Try to maintain a straight spine with your hips positioned in a way that they are supporting your spine. If you are unable to attain this position, just try to assume the most comfortable position you can. Now, with your eyes still closed, notice if your mind is quiet or if it is just running on its own. If it is running on its own, it may be the intellectual mind (where your analytical, evaluative thoughts dominate) or the emotional mind (where your thoughts about your emotional states dominate) at work. Now place your attention on your breath, first on the inhale as the air goes through your nostrils, noticing how it feels for air to slowly move into your nostrils and pass all the way into your lungs, and then on the exhale as the air is released into the atmosphere. As you continue placing your attention on your breath, actively slow your breathing down. Try to achieve about six to eight breaths per minute if you are able. Just do your best and be sure that you remain comfortable. Do not let the focus of counting breaths distract you from the goal. You will begin to notice that by simply slowing your breathing, you will start to relax and you will begin to achieve a quiet mind. Eventually, with practice, your mind will start to quiet and you will begin to drift into the overself, a state of pure observation without judgment of the thoughts passing through your awareness. Something this simple will begin to give you some sense of relief. Try to make the time taken for your inhalation the same as the time taken for your exhalation. Hold the breath for just a split second between your inhalation and your exhalation.

How often to practice: Practice this from ten to fifteen minutes twice a day if possible, or at least as often as you can.

Breathing Exercise 2

When you have slowed the rate of your breathing to the point where you have a quiet mind, begin to practice interoception. That is, begin to perceive what sensations exist inside of your body. Try to distinguish which is pain and which is a sensation of energy. They are very different in that energy has a neutral label. Also, try to let the sensations come to you instead of you seeking them. This can be achieved by attaining a quiet mind and passively observing your thoughts. Just remain present with a quiet mind and allow information from your body to enter your mind.

How often to practice: Practice this exercise every day. Performing this exercise can help prepare you for doing the more complex exercises to come.

• • •

EXERCISE 7:
HONESTY

To most people, honesty means telling the truth. For example, we can be honest with others about our thoughts and feelings, which is important. However, in order to effectively clear the burdens that we hold inside of ourselves—and which keep us in pain—we must practice *being honest with ourselves.* Honesty with ourselves means telling ourselves exactly how we feel in this moment.

Why is self-honesty important for people with chronic pain? For many, coping involves avoiding and not observing their emotions. Avoidance is a kind of dishonesty with the self, because it means we are not looking at the truths inside us. We turn away from them, often because we believe that they may be emotionally painful. This coping style of avoidance has to change in order for you to be able to observe yourself and the burden that you carry. When you begin to do this, it will bring you much more into the present moment.

Honesty Exercise

There are four steps in this exercise:
1. feeling without judgment
2. life review
3. reframing the past
4. honest acceptance without judgment

Feeling without judgment

Close your eyes and feel what is inside of your body. What you feel can be a simple sensation. Try not to give the feelings a narrative. (That is, do not give the feelings a story or an explanation.) Just be honest: This is how I feel now . . . This is how I feel at this moment . . .

Concurrent use of the slowed breathing exercise here is appropriate to help quiet the mind, which will then enable you to feel what is there—what you actually feel when you are honest.

Life review

Once you have identified your current feelings and sensations, think about your life. Has your life gone well? Are there things about your life that you would change if you were given the opportunity? If there are, how are those things affecting your present life? In order to be honest about these aspects of your life, try to avoid using judgment. Just view them as events. See them as though you were viewing a movie from a third-person perspective.

Reframing the past

After honestly and objectively reviewing the key events in your life, you can now put these events into perspective by coming to recognize that everything that has happened until this present moment cannot be changed. Thus, you have to accept all that has occurred so far. This will be a learning experience as you accept your past but release the pain attached to it. The past should no longer be a liability; it should not continue to create pain. Learning to be in the present is the best chance we have to change our future to a life without pain. This is a form of reframing what you have already learned. Reframing will help you begin to free yourself from the burden of the past that may be affecting your current life.

Honest acceptance without judgment

Now, return to just closing your eyes and allowing yourself to feel. Just be honest and begin to acknowledge the impact that the pain you experienced throughout your lifetime may have had on you. How has it influenced your present life? How has it changed your relationships with others and with yourself? How has it changed your ability to engage in life? How will it influence your future?

Remember, honesty does not have to involve judgment. Judgment sometimes brings us away from honesty. Take your time in answering these questions.

How often to practice: Practice these four steps in sequence as often as needed in order to gain a clear understanding about how pain has changed your life. Remember, honesty is extremely important in conquering pain, but honesty does not have to include judgment. This means no beating yourself up about the past. It means just viewing the events of your life as though you were watching a movie and learning and understanding. Although it will always be helpful to occasionally return to this exercise for practice, once you feel confident that you can view your pain with honesty, you should not have to do the exercise every day. Just return to it when you feel stuck and frustrated, as it will give you a clear perspective and starting point from which to improve.

•

This exercise will help you switch your attention to the future. The future is what you will begin to change.

• • •

EXERCISE 8:
WHAT DO I FEEL?

Now it is time to recognize that many feelings exist inside of your body. For the most part, people do not have access to these feelings because they have chosen not to pay attention to them or have never learned how to do so.

Feeling Sensations Exercise 1

This exercise is designed to help you feel sensations—to feel other sensations in your body besides pain and anxiety.

The exercise itself is simple. Close your eyes and use the breathing exercises (exercise 6) to slow down the rate of your breathing. Focus your attention on the inside of your chest and notice what sensations you feel. Try to allow yourself to simply feel sensations without any narrative. What you feel may be a tingling, warm, or tight feeling. You may also feel uneasiness. This is normal. Allow yourself to keep your attention focused on what you are feeling. At this point, simply feel the sensations; later, you will learn about how to feel these sensations as energy. For example, if you are in pain, feel the sensation associated with being in pain. Try to just experience the sensation in your body that is associated with pain. Place your attention on it and let it come to you. Now focus in a step-wise manner on your abdomen, then your pelvis, upper legs, knees, lower legs, and feet, taking a moment at each level to feel the sensations. Then turn your attention to your head, then your neck, and finally your arms. Practice going from head to toe, remembering to take a moment at each level to just feel sensations. At first you will probably be distracted by pain or the intellectual mind, but as you continue, you will notice that there are many other sensations inside your body besides pain.

How often to practice: Practice this exercise often (at least once a day, along with your breathing exercise—if possible, two to four times a day in the beginning) until you find that you are consciously aware of the sensations you are feeling inside your body quite regularly. Then, return to this exercise at least once or twice per week.

Up to this point, you have not given yourself permission to feel without judgment. It is time to do so.

Feeling Sensations Exercise 2: Permission to Feel

Being able to feel without judgment means that you are placing your attention on the sensations inside of you and are allowing them to remain purely sensations that are being perceived, sensations that may have elemental components but have no narrative attached. When they remain in the realm of perception, they do not have meaning or a story attached. It is important to officially tell yourself, and remind yourself, to feel sensations without attaching a narrative or judgment. Adding this to the first feeling sensation exercise gives you permission to stop the narrative, escape the judgment, and go inside of your body to feel only sensations. This one takes practice.

How often to practice: Add this exercise to the first feeling sensation exercise every day until you can perform it with confidence, and then return to it once or twice per week.

·

People who are in chronic pain become very afraid of feeling. They anticipate that every feeling is going to have a negative quality that will only make them feel worse. It is important that you recognize when you are fearful of your feelings and then give yourself permission to feel the sensations that arise within your body without fear or judgment.

• • •

EXERCISE 9:
EXTEROCEPTION VERSUS INTEROCEPTION

In this exercise, you will practice perceiving without a narrative. There are two environments from which to perceive.

Exteroception Exercise

One environment is the world outside of your body. The process of perceiving sensations from this environment is called *exteroception.* Try looking at what you see in the world around you and breaking it down into its basic elements. Observe angles, colors, and different shades. During this exercise, do not create a narrative. Try this several times throughout your day.

Interoception Exercise

The other environment is the world inside your body. The process of perceiving sensations from this environment is called *interoception.* Generally, people are very good at exteroception but are poor at interoception. It is important that you begin to practice interoception more. The only way to improve your perception skill is to practice. Make sure that you are clear that these environments are vastly different. Now that you know what exteroception is like, you will be better able to distinguish the external and internal environments with greater clarity. In this exercise, you begin to match the sensations you feel inside of your body with your emotions. You may begin to realize that these emotions predated any physical pain. You are likely to also discover that *not* feeling these sensations and the attached emotions can contribute significantly to suffering.

First allow yourself to feel sensations inside your body, and then allow the associated narrative to come into your mind. Begin to observe the narrative as though you were watching a movie—that is, watch from the *I*-the-perceiver, or "objective self" perspective. Explore the first time you felt the emotion related to the sensation. Then return to the sensation itself. Next, explore other times you have felt the same sensation. Attempt to remain without judgment throughout this exercise. Simply watch the movie and feel the sensations.

For example, let's say you begin to feel sensations in either your abdomen or your chest and begin to break those sensations down into their elemental parts. You may notice an emotion associated with the sensations. Now ask yourself, "When was the first time I felt that emotion?" If a narrative comes into your mind, pay attention to the narrative. Then place your attention back on the sensations. Feel free to ask yourself the question, "When was the first time I felt those sensations?" Then ask yourself, "When were some other times that I felt those sensations?" Do this without analysis, evaluation, or judgment. Let the information come to you. Emotion experienced this way may be thought of as sensation with a narrative.

How often to practice: Practice this exercise every day to prepare yourself for learning how to clear sensations that you have internalized and that are likely associated with burden.

•

This is the end of the first set of exercises. Please feel confident in these exercises before you continue on to the more complex exercises. Exercises 1 through 9 can bring you a significant amount of relief from your chronic pain. Before we begin with the second set of exercises, we will take some time in the following section to bring together what we have learned so far and explore what it means to achieve the balance that is essential to preventing chronic pain from recurring.

• • •

Balance

Taking steps to find balance in your life is important. When your life was consumed by pain, you may have lost the ability to have balance and to carry out healthy routines, or routines may be things that you never really learned to create. Living in a balanced way means that you lower your stress level and learn how to keep it minimized, you get enough rest, you eat well, you move in a mindful manner, you do mindfulness exercises, and your mind has periods of quiet. These periods of quiet mind should be increasing every day, and you should be actively working to increase the frequency of your experience of quiet mind. This can be done by simply getting into a routine that enables you to start doing healthy things and reducing stress. Again, it is important that you begin to experience balance and healthy routines, whether for the first time in your life or as something you are regaining.

Developing a Routine that Increases Balance

Besides practicing breathing exercises, your routine to achieve balance should include getting adequate sleep, eating in a healthy way, and practicing some form of gentle exercise.

Sleep. Begin to practice a routine in the evening in which you are able to calm your mind enough so that you fall asleep, and if you awaken in stress, you are able to go back to that calm state. This can begin with exercise 6 (Breathing): simply pay attention to your inhalations and exhalations.

Nutrition. Eating in a healthy manner is important. You should eat small portions, enough to satisfy your hunger, and do not skip meals. Avoid binge eating. Eat a well-balanced diet, and avoid excess amounts of sugar and fat. Consult with your primary care physician, or a nutritionist, for your specific dietary needs.

Gentle physical exercise. In the next set of exercises, we will talk about the importance of movement, such as taking a Qigong, tai chi, or yoga class. These classes can help you learn to move easily and can also help you establish a pleasant routine that you can continue once the class has ended. Regardless of which type of movement you choose, begin to move and stretch daily.

The next exercise comes just before the more complex exercises that help you view and move energy.

. . .

EXERCISE 10:

MOVEMENT

People with chronic pain often restrict their movements, though as I noted earlier in this book, they are often surprised to learn just how much they do move. As part of your recovery, it is important that you begin to move. This movement should be mindful and, at first, very gentle.

Movement Exercise 1

People with chronic pain do not remember how to move their muscles in a normal way. You must regain the memory of what it feels like for muscles to function normally and for the body to move normally. That is the purpose of this exercise.

Mindful movement is movement in which you place attention on how your body is moving from moment to moment. If there are particular areas of your body that hurt, place your attention on those areas and then very gently start to move them. Your movements should be very gentle and slow, either back and forth or moving in one direction and gently stretching. Begin to notice if any of your movements are restricted. If there are restrictions, do everything you can to overcome those restrictions. For example, if you have headaches and there appears to be no way to move your neck, begin by slowly and gently moving the muscles of your shoulders, the muscles in the back of your neck, or the muscles in the front of your neck and determine if you are holding stress in those areas.

There are two things to pay attention to when you are moving your muscles. First, are the muscles in spasm? When muscles are in spasm, it means they are tightened. If this is the case, you need to stretch them gently and move them slowly. Second, are the muscles holding tension and emotion? This feels different from spasm and tightness. If you carefully set your hand on the muscles and they automatically hurt with even this gentle touch, then you are holding emotions and stress. Gently start to move the affected muscles and allow yourself to begin to relieve the emotions and stress. When you begin this exercise, be very gentle on yourself. It is going to take time to move muscles that have not been moved in a while. If possible, consult a health care professional or work with an instructor in a yoga, tai chi, or Qigong class. Nevertheless, please begin to move.

Also, remember that exercise should have a mindful component—that is, it should allow you to be in the present moment and not held captive by the past or future. Just be in the moment as the breath comes in and out of your lungs.

How often to practice: You should practice this exercise every day, and remember to do it very gently at first. When you do this exercise, make sure that you place your attention on different areas and eventually try to move every muscle in your body. At first, the movement may be limited to simply flexing the muscle. You must remember to do this exercise every day.

Movement Exercise 2

You have already begun to move gently. Now it is time to begin adding more energy to your movement. However, you must do so in a mindful manner—movement without judgment, with attention to your inner sensations, and with a quiet mind. Structured, or more formal, movement is conducive to achieving mindfulness while moving.

If available, join a reputable Qigong class or follow the recommendations for finding reputable Qigong instruction materials in exercise 12, Qigong. The point is for you to move your body in a mindful manner and do more active and formal movement than you practiced in the first movement exercise. Whichever movement practice you adopt, do it mindfully. You will learn more about how to do this in exercise 12. Qigong is movement that is mindful, has a purpose, and is healing. This will be a key practice for learning to experience and move energy.

How often to practice: Practice at least three times a week or as often as time permits.

•

The next group of exercises is more advanced and should be practiced after you feel confident with exercises 1 through 10.

• • •

EXERCISE 11:
INTRODUCTION TO ENERGY

In the practice of Qigong, one uses the breath, energy, and movement to achieve a quiet mind. There are two types of movement involved: (1) the movement of the muscles and joints of the body and (2) the movement of Qi, the energy of life.

Introduction to Energy Exercise

This exercise will help you develop the ability to observe energy within your body. In subsequent exercises, you will use this ability to allow your body to heal itself.

Close your eyes and begin to slow your breathing. Place your attention on the sensations inside of your body. These sensations are a form of energy. They may feel like tingling or heat. If you do not notice feeling anything at first, it is okay. If you are trying hard and seeking information, remember to be patient and let the information come to you. Remember also to apply the honesty you practiced in exercise 7. If nothing happens, do not try to manufacture something—just be honest with yourself about what you are experiencing. Try slowing the rate of your breathing and allow the information to appear.

As you observe the energy, notice the quality of your experience. Do you feel tingling or heat? Does your consciousness perceive light or darkness? Do you experience a particular color in your consciousness? You may notice many different types of experiences as you allow yourself to observe energy. Simply notice them without creating a narrative, and continue the process.

When you try to view energy, it is important that you remain passive. You should simply have the intention of watching the energy. If you try to seek the energy, nothing will appear. This practice is about simply having the intention of viewing or observing the energy. When I do this exercise with patients, I always tell them, "Do not seek. Do not want. Be thankful for whatever you are given in this process and much more will come your way." In other words, what comes is a gift because you are tuning in to your ability to heal.

214

You must understand that the body already has the ability to heal. The body is equipped with a mechanism to heal. The body has a consciousness. Remember, quiet the mind and then simply have the intention to heal. Have the intention to observe energy inside of your body. Energy may take on a visual aspect or a tactile aspect or both. Just practice observing.

How often to practice: Ideally, you should practice observing energy every day for the rest of your life.

• • •

EXERCISE 12:

QIGONG

The healing force of Qigong is Qi, or the energy of life. It is now appropriate to adjust your perspective of the body from a strictly mechanical and material viewpoint and begin to view your body as a field of energy. In order to do so, it will be necessary to do exercises that help you develop this skill.

Qigong exercise, or what is referred to as internal Qigong, will help you to cultivate energy. Strengthening your sense of internal energy improves your ability to use energy to heal yourself. Again, I must emphasize that this is a much different perspective from other healing methods. By regularly performing Qigong exercises, you will learn how to build energy, quiet the mind, and use the breath to gain health. You will heal if you routinely practice the exercises. It does not help to try to analyze them or understand them in a linear fashion.

Qigong Exercise

It is beyond the scope of this book to present a full set of formal Qigong exercises. I suggest you visit the website for the Qigong Institute, www.qigonginstitute.org, where you will find a number of resources, instructional videos, and recommendations for DVDs and books for beginners through advanced practitioners.

One book that I recommend is *Qigong Empowerment: A Guide to Medical, Taoist, Buddhist, and Wushu Energy Cultivation* by Master Shou-Yu Liang and Wen-Ching Wu. Another more accessible and popular book is *The Way of Qigong: The Art and Science of Chinese Energy Healing* by Kenneth S. Cohen.

There are many different schools and forms of Qigong. All that you need to do is watch the exercises on the Qigong Institute website or one of the recommended DVDs (there are also several exercises available on YouTube) or follow the instructions in one of the books and then pick one or more with which you feel comfortable, try them out, and begin to practice the exercises to the best of your ability. Practice every day. If it is easier to just take three or four exercises and repeat them, feel free to do that. Be gentle on yourself and do not judge and evaluate yourself. Every step is important. This is not about "pushing through."

Another option is to sign up for a formal Qigong class. This would be best, if you have the ability to do so.

The most important thing is that you have the intention to heal. Nothing else will be as important.

How often to practice: Ideally, Qigong would become a practice that you incorporate into your daily life. But I understand many are limited by time, so do this practice as often as you can.

· · ·

EXERCISE 13:
VIEWING ENERGY

By doing this Qigong exercise of viewing energy, you will learn how to build energy, quiet the mind, and use the breath to gain health.

Viewing Energy Exercise

When you view energy, you simply allow the information to come to you. The entry point can be placing your attention on your breathing and slowing your breath. This is something that you have practiced before, in exercise 6, so it is not new. After you have slowed your breathing to a steady rate of approximately six to eight breaths per minute, begin to place your attention inside of your body. You may want to begin in one area, such as your abdomen, or view your body in its entirety. When you view energy, just focus your attention inside of your body and hold the intention of being aware and passively observing without judgment. Passive observation involves allowing information to come to you without actively seeking. It will take time to understand this, but when you have gained the ability to have a quiet mind, this type of observation will be much easier. You must not have any expectancy—whatever happens when you are doing this exercise is okay. Allow your body, mind, brain, and spirit to do the work. Whatever information you receive is appropriate. Do not judge; do not seek; do not want something to happen. Just allow energy to come your way. Simply observe the information inside of you.

How often to practice: Ideally, this would become a daily lifetime practice, but perform it as often as you can.

• • •

EXERCISE 14:
PERSPECTIVE

This exercise is designed to help you realize that you have taken a new perspective. You are now viewing the information inside of your body as energy. Although this is new and may not be easy at first, it will soon enable you to transform yourself.

Perspective Exercise

This exercise will begin to teach you to observe and build energy.

As you slow the rate of your breathing and balance the rhythm of your breath (inhalation matches exhalation), assume the perspective of being inside one of your lungs and viewing air as it enters. Watch the air come into your lungs. Understand that the air carries oxygen and the oxygen passes through tissue in your lungs, goes into the blood, and is carried to every other tissue throughout the body. When the oxygen reaches the tissues, it creates energy. You can imagine that as the oxygen crosses your lungs and goes into your blood, it is creating energy.

Sit quietly and imagine this process occurring. At first, just place your attention on the air coming into your lungs and being carried to every tissue of your body. Then, start to feel the energy that is building in your hands, in your feet, and throughout the rest of your body.

It is good to practice this for ten to twenty minutes at a time. Remember that as the air passes through your lungs, it is creating energy. It is building energy. Allow yourself to view this process as the energy builds.

How often to practice: Practice this every day along with the breathing exercise for the first four weeks. Thereafter, it will become part of another exercise.

• • •

EXERCISE 15:
ADVERSITY CONFRONTED AND CLEARED

After you have practiced exercises 13 and 14 and learned to view sensations in your body as energy, it is time to begin clearing out the negative energy that is creating a burden inside your body. This exercise explains how this process works.

Clearing Adversity Exercise

This exercise will teach you how to clear the negative energy that is trapped inside of you and creating adversity.

This exercise builds on what you learned in exercise 14, Perspective, where you observed the energy in your lungs. As you begin to slow the rate of your breathing and view energy in your body, you will notice that some areas seem to be trapping or holding negative energy. Ask yourself when you first felt that energy and observe if any narrative comes into your mind. Simply allow the narrative to pass. As it begins to pass, continue to keep your attention on the energy. Now focus your attention on the breath. Imagine that as the air comes into your lungs, it is merging with the energy. If you allow it to merge, your breath will carry the energy. You can then feel this negative energy clear from your body with each slow exhalation and continue to release after the exhalation is completed until the energy has dissipated. Through this process, you are clearing the adversity, held as stagnant energy, from your body. At first, this may take some practice.

How often to practice: This exercise should now become the focus of your practice and performed daily in addition to movement and mindfulness.

• • •

EXERCISE 16:
FIVE GATEWAYS

Now that you have begun to observe energy, I will describe five areas inside of your body from which you can observe energy. Observing your energy from these areas will allow you to build and create energy.

Five Gateways Exercise

Through this exercise you will learn to observe energy, to cultivate energy, and to move while allowing energy to heal your body.

When you begin these exercises, always begin with slowing the rate of your breathing and then finding a safe place inside of your lungs from which you can observe energy in your body (exercise 14). As you begin to observe the exchange of oxygen passing into your blood and building energy, you can try observing your energy from five areas (five gateways).

Gateway one: Go from your lungs up to your head and find the bridge of your nose. Now go one finger width up from the bridge of your nose and two finger widths inside of your head. Observe energy from this perspective.

Gateway two: Go from your lungs slightly to the left until you feel you are at your heart; then go two finger widths to the right. This is the next area from which you can observe energy.

Gateway three: From the center of your chest, go down to the end of your ribs where your diaphragm attaches. Then go two finger widths underneath. This is the next area from which you can observe energy.

Gateway four: From the center of your chest, go all the way down into your upper abdomen. Find your navel at the center. At the end of the navel, go three finger widths below the navel. This is the next area from which you can observe energy.

Gateway five: Go all the way down to the tops of your feet and then to the end of the tops of your feet. Follow along the center of your big toes until you come to the end. Now go to the bottoms of your big toes and follow along the center until it ends; then follow the center of the balls of your feet until they end. At the ends of the balls of your feet, travel two finger widths back. This is the next area from which you can observe energy.

As you observe energy from each of these gateways, remember to allow the information to come to you. Do not seek. Do not want. Whatever you are given is what is appropriate for you to observe at the time. Simply have the intention of observing without judgment or expectation, and be thankful for what comes your way.

How often to practice: Practice this exercise three times per week.

• • •

EXERCISE 17:
EMOTIONS PROCESSED

In exercise 15, you learned how to use the breath to clear negative energy associated with past emotional experiences that have been internalized. Now that you have been practicing viewing the inside of your body as energy, you are ready to move that energy and allow it to heal.

Processing Internalized Emotions as Energy Exercise

This practice will allow you to move energy and heal.

When you reach the point where you feel comfortable doing exercise 16, Five Gateways, you will begin to notice areas inside your body that may be holding negative energy. Now allow yourself to move that energy. The body knows how to do this. You do not have to try hard or make a conscious effort. It just takes intention. *Intention* means placing yourself in the mindset that you want to heal and you will not try to control the healing process. Place your attention on the energy and then allow the energy to move. It is as simple as that: you intend for the energy to move. You do not try to make it move.

How often to practice: Now that you have reached this stage in the exercises, this exercise becomes your focus. If you need to go back and review any of the other exercises, feel free to do so, as they are the foundation for practicing exercise 17. Exercise 15 can be viewed as a similar exercise, since both involve processing burden, adversity, and negative emotional energy.

• • •

EXERCISE 18:
CONSCIOUSNESS

Quieting the mind to achieve a sense of consciousness is still probably a new and challenging experience, but the more you practice, the easier it will become. Understand that just as the mind has an intelligence, the body has an intelligence, but the intelligence of the body is not at all like that of the mind. The intelligence of the body allows your newly discovered consciousness to gather information in a new way. It is passive because you do not have to try. The information simply comes to you. All that is necessary is that you are present and willing to allow information to come your way. All you need to do is have the intention to let your body heal. This is simple, though we tend to make it difficult.

Consciousness Exercise

This exercise will help you maintain a healing consciousness.

Take a moment to reflect on the previous exercises. Which ones seem most helpful for you in achieving a quiet mind? When you have time during the day, allow yourself to enter into a quiet mind, to stop making judgments, and to allow yourself to have the intention to heal. Do not try; just allow it to occur.

As you allow your mind to be quiet, you will learn more about your consciousness. Simply allow the information to come to you. That is how the body's intelligence works. All you have to do is be present and have a quiet mind. Do nothing else; all the information you need is there and will come to you.

How often to practice: Practice this exercise as often as you can each day.

•

It is important at this stage that you get into a daily routine of practicing any of these eighteen exercises that you find most helpful. I am hopeful that you have arrived at a place where you can perceive energy, perhaps move energy, and clear energy that is associated with the burden that you have internalized. No matter how much, or how little, time you have during your day, try to do some exercises and allow energy to move. These practices can become a part of your lifestyle. They will help you relieve yourself from pain and burden.

. . .

Conclusion:
Retraining Mind and Body

We have come to the end of the exercises, and the end of the book. In the first part of this book, you learned about your brain, your mind, and your body. The second part contained exercises designed to help you conquer chronic pain. The first part of this book acts on your intellectual and emotional minds. In the exercises, you learned to escape the intellectual and emotional minds. Success happens through practice—practice that alters the structure of your brain, changes the way your mind works, helps you discover the overself, helps you release the burdens of past pain and adversity, and allows your body's natural healing ability to reach its full potential and be realized.

To retrain your brain, mind, and body, you must practice. Please ask yourself if you are willing to commit time *each day* to practicing these exercises so you can relieve yourself from the burden of chronic pain. Will you commit to a lifestyle of balance and health? These exercises can bring you to that end. Please commit to *do something* every day.

You have spent years, perhaps much of your life, suffering. Give yourself permission to be relieved from this suffering. You are not meant to suffer. No one is. With that in mind, here is one final exercise for you:

Stop suffering

How often to practice: Every minute of the rest of your life.

How to do it: Practice these exercises. Stop judgment. Begin a balanced life. Allow yourself to heal.

. . .

References

American Academy of Pain Medicine, The. *AAPM facts and figures on pain.* Retrieved from www.painmed.org/patientcenter/facts_on_pain.aspx

Banta, J. E., Haviland, M. G., & Przekop, P. (2008). Datapoints: Mapping estimated county-level income and binge drinking among California men. *Psychiatric Services, 59*(2), 138.

Banta, J. E., Przekop, P., Haviland, M. G., & Pereau, M. (2008). Binge drinking among California adults: Results from the 2005 California Health Interview Survey. *The American Journal of Drug and Alcohol Abuse, 34,* 801–809. Erratum in: (2009). *The American Journal of Drug and Alcohol Abuse, 35,* 203.

Beckett, A. H. & Casey, A. F. (1954). Synthetic analgesics: Stereochemical considerations. *Journal of Pharmacology, 6,* 986–1001.

Brunton, P. (1937). *The quest of the overself.* The Random House Group.

Centers for Disease Control and Prevention. (2011, November 1). *Prescription painkiller overdoses at epidemic levels: Kill more Americans than heroin and cocaine combined.* Retrieved from www.cdc.gov/media/releases/2011/p1101_flu _pain_killer_overdose.html

Centers for Disease Control and Prevention. (2013, July 5). Vital signs: Overdoses of prescription opioid pain relievers and other drugs among women—United States, 1999–2010. *Morbidity and Mortality Weekly Report 62*(26), 537–542.

Centers for Disease Control and Prevention. (2014, July 1). Opioid painkiller prescribing varies widely among states: Where you live makes a difference. Retrieved from www.cdc.gov/media/releases/2014/p0701-opioid-painkiller .html

Centers for Disease Control and Prevention. (2015, April 30). *Prescription drug overdose data.* Retrieved from www.cdc.gov/drugoverdose/data/overdose .html

Cohen, K. S. (1999). *The way of Qigong: The art and science of Chinese energy healing.* New York, NY: Wellspring/Ballantine.

Committee on Advancing Pain Research, Care, and Education, Board on Health Sciences Policy, & Institute of Medicine of the National Academies. (2011). *Relieving pain in America: A blueprint for transforming prevention, care, education, and research.* Washington, DC: The National Academies Press.

Franklin, G. M. (2014, September 30). Opioids for chronic noncancer pain: A position paper of the American Academy of Neurology. *Neurology 83*(14), 1277–1284.

Haskard, K. B., Banta, J. E., Williams, S. L., Haviland, M. G., DiMatteo, M. R., Przekop, P., Werner, L. S., & Anderson, D. L. (2008). Binge drinking, poor mental health, and adherence to treatment among California adults with asthma. *Journal of Asthma, 45,* 369–376.

Haviland, M. G., Banta, J. E., & Przekop, P. (2011). Fibromyalgia: Prevalence, course, and co-morbidities in hospitalized patients in the United States, 1999–2007. *Clinical and Experimental Rheumatology, 29* (6, Suppl. 69), S79–87.

Haviland, M. G., Banta, J. E., & Przekop, P. (2011, September). *Hospitalization charges for fibromyalgia in the United States, 1999–2007.* Poster session presented at the meeting of the American Academy of Pain Management, Las Vegas, NV.

Haviland, M. G., Banta, J. E., & Przekop, P. (2012). Hospitalization charges for fibromyalgia in the United States, 1999–2007. *Clinical and Experimental Rheumatology, 30* (6, Suppl. 74), S129–135.

Haviland, M. G., Przekop, P., Oda, K., & Morton, K. R. (2012, September). *Pain interference in the lives of older adults.* Poster session presented at the meeting of the American Academy of Pain Management, Phoenix, AZ.

Hebb, D. (1949). *The organization of behavior: A Neuropsychological theory.* New York, NY: Wiley & Sons.

Hill, D. L., & Przekop, P. R. (1988, September). Influence of dietary sodium on functional taste receptor development: A sensitive period. *Science, 241*(4874), 1826–1828.

Johannes, C. B., Le, T. K., Zhou, X., Johnston, J. A., & Dworkin, R. H. (2010). The prevalence of chronic pain in United States adults: Results of an Internet-based survey. *Journal of Pain, 11*(11). Retrieved from www.ncbi.nlm .nih.gov/pubmed/20797916

Koch, C. (2004). *The quest for consciousness: A neurobiological approach.* Greenwood Village, CO: Roberts and Company Publishers.

Lenneberg, E. H. (1967). *Biological foundations of language.* Hoboken, NJ: John Wiley & Sons.

Liang, S. & Wu, W. (1996). *Qigong empowerment: A guide to medical, Taoist, Buddhist, and Wushu energy cultivation.* East Providence, RI: The Way of the Dragon Publishing.

Luria A. R. (1966). *Higher cortical functions in man.* Basic Books.

Lutz, P., & Kieffer, B. L. (2013, March). Opioid receptors: Distinct roles in mood disorders. *Trends in Neuroscience, 36*(3), 195–206.

Maguire, E. A., Woollett, K., & Spiers, H. J. (2006). London taxi drivers and bus drivers: A structural MRI and neuropsychological analysis. *Hippocampus 16,* 1091–1101.

Pert, C. B., & Snyder, S. H. (1973). Properties of opiate-receptor binding in rat brain. *Proceedings of the National Academy of Sciences of the United States of America, 70*(8), 2243–2247.

Portenoy, R. K. (2013). Risks associated with opioid use. *JAMA, 310*(16), 1738.

Przekop, P., Haviland, M. G., Morton, K. R., Oda, K., & Fraser, G.E. (2010). Correlates of perceived pain-related restrictions among women with fibromyalgia. *Pain Medicine, 11,* 1698–1706.

Przekop, P., Haviland, M. G., Oda, K., & Morton, K. R. (2014). Prevalence and correlates of pain interference in older adults: Why treating the whole body and mind is necessary. *Journal of Bodywork & Movement Therapies.* Advance online publication. doi: 10.1016/j.jbmt.2014.04.011

Przekop, P., Haviland, M. G., Zhao, Y., Oda, K., Morton, K. R., & Fraser, G.E. (2011, September). *Perceived physical and mental health and co-morbid diseases among women with irritable bowel syndrome, fibromyalgia, neither, or both disorders.* Poster session presented at the meeting of the American Academy of Pain Management, Las Vegas, NV.

Przekop, P., Haviland, M. G., Zhao, Y., Oda, K., Morton, K. R., & Fraser, G. E. (2012). Perceived physical and mental health and co-morbid diseases among women with irritable bowel syndrome, fibromyalgia, neither, or both disorders. *Journal of the American Osteopathic Association, 112,* 726–735. Erratum in: (2013). *Journal of the American Osteopathic Association, 113,* 15.

Przekop, P., Przekop, A., Ashwal, S., Haviland, M. G., & Riggs, M. L. (2009, April). *Neurocognitive enhancement for the treatment of chronic nonmalignant pain.* Paper presented at the meeting of the American Academy of Neurology, Seattle, WA.

Przekop, P., Przekop, A., & Haviland, M. G. (2012, September). *Preventive strategy for pediatric migraine headache.* Poster session presented at the meeting of the American Academy of Pain Management, Phoenix, AZ.

Przekop, P., Przekop, A., & Haviland, M. G. (2013, September). *Pharmacologic and non-pharmacologic treatments of adolescents with chronic tension-type headache.* Poster session presented at the meeting of the American Academy of Pain Management, Orlando, FL.

Przekop, P., Przekop, A., & Haviland, M. G. (2014, May). *Pharmacologic and non-pharmacologic treatments of adolescents with chronic tension-type headache.* Poster session presented at the meeting of the American Academy of Neurology, Philadelphia, PA.

Przekop, P., Przekop, A., & Haviland, M. G. (2015). Multimodal compared to pharmacologic treatments for chronic tension-type headache in adolescents. Accepted *Journal of Bodywork & Movement Therapies.*

Przekop P., Przekop A., & Haviland M. G. (2015, April). *Comparisons of patients with non-cancer pain taking and not taking chronic opioid therapy.* Poster session presented at the meeting of the American Academy of Neurology, Washington, DC.

Przekop, P., Przekop, A., Haviland, M. G., & Riggs, M. L. (2009, May). *Neurocognitive enhancement for the treatment of chronic pain in chemically dependent patients.* Paper presented at the meeting of the American Society of Addiction Medicine, New Orleans, LA.

Przekop, P., Przekop, A., Haviland, M. G., & Riggs, M. L. (2010). Neurocognitive enhancement for the treatment of chronic pain [Fascia Congress Abstract]. *Journal of Bodywork & Movement Therapies, 14,* 334–335.

Przekop, P. R., Mook, D. G., & Hill, D. L. (1990, October). Functional recovery of the gustatory system after sodium deprivation during development: how much sodium and where? *American Journal of Physiology, 259*(4), R786–791.

Raichle, M. E., MacLeod, A. M., Snyder, A. Z., Powers, W. J., Gusnard, D. A., & Shulman, G. L. (2011, January 16). A default mode of brain function. *Proceedings of the National Academy of Sciences of the United States of America 98*(2): 676–682.

Ricks, D. (January 21, 2012). UN: U.S. consumes 80% of world's oxycodone. *Newsday.* Retrieved from www.newsday.com/news/health/un-u-s-consumes -80-of-world-s-oxycodone-1.3469762

Rosenblatt, R. A,, & Catlin, M. (2012). Opioids for chronic pain: First do no harm. *Annals of Family Medicine 10*(4): 300–301.

Searle, J. R. (1997, September) *The mystery of consciousness.* New York, NY: The New York Review of Books.

Seminowicz, D. A., Wideman, T. H., Naso, L., Hatami-Khoroushahi, Z., Fallatah, S., Ware, M. A., Jarzem, P., Bushnell, M. C., Shir, Y., Ouellet, J. A., & Stone, L. S. (2011, May 18). Effective treatment of chronic low back pain in humans reverses abnormal brain anatomy and function. *The Journal of Neuroscience 31*(20), 7540–7550.

Weinstein, J. N., Lurie, J. D., Olson, P., Bronner, K. K., Fisher, E. S., & Morgan, T. S. (2006, November 1). United States trends and regional variations in lumbar spine surgery: 1992–2003. *Spine, 31*(23), 2707–2714.

Wick, B., Przekop, P., & Haviland, M. G. (2008, May). *The psychosocial burden of chronic pain.* Poster session presented at the meeting of the American Psychiatric Association, Washington, DC.

About the Author

Peter Przekop, DO, PhD, has been doing research and developing his alternative model for managing chronic pain for over ten years, four of them with the chronic pain clinic at the Betty Ford Center, and has published a number of research papers on the subject.

• • •

About Hazelden Publishing

As part of the Hazelden Betty Ford Foundation, Hazelden Publishing offers both cutting-edge educational resources and inspirational books. Our print and digital works help guide individuals in treatment and recovery, and their loved ones. Professionals who work to prevent and treat addiction also turn to Hazelden Publishing for evidence-based curricula, digital content solutions, and videos for use in schools, treatment programs, correctional programs, and electronic health records systems. We also offer training for implementation of our curricula.

Through published and digital works, Hazelden Publishing extends the reach of healing and hope to individuals, families, and communities affected by addiction and related issues.

For more information about Hazelden publications,
please call **800-328-9000**
or visit us online at **hazelden.org/bookstore.**

• • •

Other Titles That May Interest You

When Painkillers Become Dangerous
What Everyone Needs to Know About OxyContin and Other Prescription Drugs
DREW PINSKY, MD, MARV SEPPALA, MD, ROBERT MYERS, PHD,
JOHN GARDIN, PHD, WILLIAM WHITE, MA, AND STEPHANIE BROWN, PHD

Best-selling author Drew Pinsky, MD, and five other leading experts offer practical, plainspoken, and much-needed information about addiction to painkilling drugs.

Order No. 2139 (softcover), EB2139 (e-book)

Pain-Free Living for Drug-Free People
A Guide to Pain Management in Recovery
MARVIN D. SEPPALA, MD, AND DAVID P. MARTIN, MD, PHD

Pain-Free Living for Drug-Free People is an information-packed guide to pain management in recovery and other issues related to pain control and addiction.

Order No. 7384 (softcover), EB7384 (e-book)

Painkillers, Heroin, and the Road to Sanity
Real Solutions for Long-Term Recovery from Opiate Addiction
JOANI GAMMILL, RN, BRII

In *Painkillers, Heroin, and the Road to Sanity,* recovering addict and prominent interventionist Joani Gammill offers a radically effective approach for those struggling with opioid addiction, sharing sometimes-controversial tips that have worked for some people in long-term recovery.

Order No. 7535 (softcover), EB7535

Hazelden Publishing books are available at fine bookstores everywhere.

To order from Hazelden Publishing, call **800-328-9000**
or visit **hazelden.org/bookstore.**